Is Stem Cell Research Necessary?

**Lauri S. Friedman
and Hal Marcovitz**

INCONTROVERSY

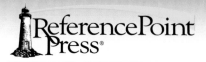

ReferencePoint
Press®

San Diego, CA

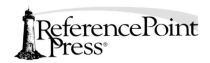

About the Authors:

Lauri S. Friedman earned her bachelor's degree in religion and political science from Vassar College in 1999. She is the founder of LSF Editorial, a writing and editing shop in San Diego. Her clients include ReferencePoint Press, for whom she has written *The Death Penalty, Nuclear Weapons and Security, Terrorist Attacks, Abortion, Islam, Assisted Suicide,* and *Fossil Fuels,* all in the Compact Research series. Friedman lives in San Diego with her husband, Randy, and their yellow lab, Trucker.

Hal Marcovitz is a former newspaper reporter who has written more than 130 books for young readers. He lives in Chalfont, Pennsylvania, with his wife, Gail, and daughter, Ashley.

Picture credits:
Cover: iStockphoto.com
Maury Aaseng: 25, 59, 78
AP Images: 7, 29
Landov: 8, 41, 54, 75
Photoshot: 36, 67
Science Photo Library: 13, 32, 62

LIBRARY OF CONGRESS CATALOGING-IN-PUBLICATION DATA

Friedman, Lauri S., and Marcovitz, Hal
  Is stem cell research necessary? / by Lauri S. Friedman and Hal Marcovitz.
     p. cm. — (In controversy)
  Includes bibliographical references and index.
  ISBN-13: 978-1-60152-088-3 (hardback)
  ISBN-10: 1-60152-088-3 (hardback)
  1. Stem cells—Research—Popular works. I. Marcovitz, Hal. II. Title.
  QH588.S83.F75 2009
  174.2'8—dc22
                                                                2009016494

Contents

Foreword   4

Introduction
Stem Cell Research: The Moral Debate   6

Chapter One
What Are the Origins of the Stem
Cell Controversy?   11

Chapter Two
What Benefits Could Stem Cell Research Offer?   24

Chapter Three
Should Scientific Promise Outweigh
Moral Concerns?   39

Chapter Four
Are There Effective Alternatives to Embryonic
Stem Cell Research?   53

Chapter Five
Should the Government Support Stem
Cell Research?   66

Related Organizations   80
For Further Research   85
Source Notes   87
Index   94

Foreword

In 2008, as the U.S. economy and economies worldwide were falling into one of the worst recessions in modern history, most Americans had difficulty comprehending the complexity, magnitude, and scope of what was happening. As is often the case with a complex, controversial issue such as this historic global economic recession, looking at the problem as a whole can be overwhelming and often does not lead to understanding. One way to better comprehend such a large issue or event is to break it into smaller parts. The intricacies of global economic recession may be difficult to understand, but one can gain insight by instead beginning with an individual contributing factor such as the real estate market. When examined through a narrower lens, complex issues become clearer and easier to evaluate.

This is the idea behind ReferencePoint Press's *In Controversy* series. The series examines the complex, controversial issues of the day by breaking them into smaller pieces. Rather than looking at the stem cell research debate as a whole, a title would examine an important aspect of the debate such as *Is Stem Cell Research Necessary?* or *Is Embryonic Stem Cell Research Ethical?* By studying the central issues of the debate individually, researchers gain a more solid and focused understanding of the topic as a whole.

Each book in the series provides a clear, insightful discussion of the issues, integrating facts and a variety of contrasting opinions for a solid, balanced perspective. Personal accounts and direct quotes from academic and professional experts, advocacy groups, politicians, and others enhance the narrative. Sidebars add depth to the discussion by expanding on important ideas and events. For quick reference, a list of key facts concludes every chapter. Source notes, an annotated organizations list, bibliography, and index provide student researchers with additional tools for papers and class discussion.

The *In Controversy* series also challenges students to think critically about issues, to improve their problem-solving skills, and to sharpen their ability to form educated opinions. As President Barack Obama stated in a March 2009 speech, success in the twenty-first century will not be measurable merely by students' ability to "fill in a bubble on a test but whether they possess 21st century skills like problem-solving and critical thinking and entrepreneurship and creativity." Those who possess these skills will have a strong foundation for whatever lies ahead.

No one can know for certain what sort of world awaits today's students. What we can assume, however, is that those who are inquisitive about a wide range of issues; open-minded to divergent views; aware of bias and opinion; and able to reason, reflect, and reconsider will be best prepared for the future. As the international development organization Oxfam notes, "Today's young people will grow up to be the citizens of the future: but what that future holds for them is uncertain. We can be quite confident, however, that they will be faced with decisions about a wide range of issues on which people have differing, contradictory views. If they are to develop as global citizens all young people should have the opportunity to engage with these controversial issues."

In Controversy helps today's students better prepare for tomorrow. An understanding of the complex issues that drive our world and the ability to think critically about them are essential components of contributing, competing, and succeeding in the twenty-first century.

Stem Cell Research: The Moral Debate

Michael J. Fox shot to stardom playing the role of Marty McFly in the movie *Back to the Future*, which tells the story of a teenager who travels back in time to make sure his parents meet at a high school dance. After starring in the film and its sequels, Fox went on to a career in TV and the movies that established him as one of the most popular actors in Hollywood.

But Fox takes few roles today. In 1991, at the age of 30, he was diagnosed with Parkinson's disease, a debilitating neurological disorder that manifests itself in slowed and slurred speech, muscle tremors, and rigid muscles. The disorder is caused by a lack of nerve cells, or neurons, in the brain that produce dopamine, a chemical that carries messages from cell to cell. Research has shown that the brain contains many more neurons than it actually needs—it is nature's way of preserving cognitive abilities as people grow older and lose brain cells during the normal process of aging. In Parkinson's disease, the cells die much more quickly, which means less dopamine is produced by the brain, leaving relatively young people fewer neurons than they need to maintain normal cognitive abilities. At first Fox was able to continue working because his symptoms were minor. But over the years his

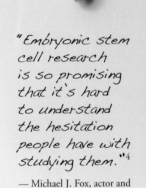

"*Embryonic stem cell research is so promising that it's hard to understand the hesitation people have with studying them.*"[4]

— Michael J. Fox, actor and Parkinson's disease patient.

symptoms have progressed, and now whenever Fox makes a public appearance, the physical tremors that make him tremble and slur his speech are evident.

A controversial process that involves the use of what are known as stem cells may hold a lot of promise for Parkinson's patients and others who suffer from cell-related diseases. During the past few years, Fox has emerged as a major proponent of stem cell research and has even established a foundation to raise money for the research. He has also called on the federal government to make billions of dollars a year available for stem cell research. Says Fox, "I really believe in the promise of stem cell research."[1]

Destroying Embryos

Stem cells can be injected into a patient, where they are believed capable of growing into normal and healthy tissue, replacing cells that are diseased or destroyed. Proponents of stem cell research

Actor Michael J. Fox, speaking at a conference in 2008, was diagnosed with Parkinson's disease at the age of 30. He believes that stem cell research offers promise for a cure for Parkinson's.

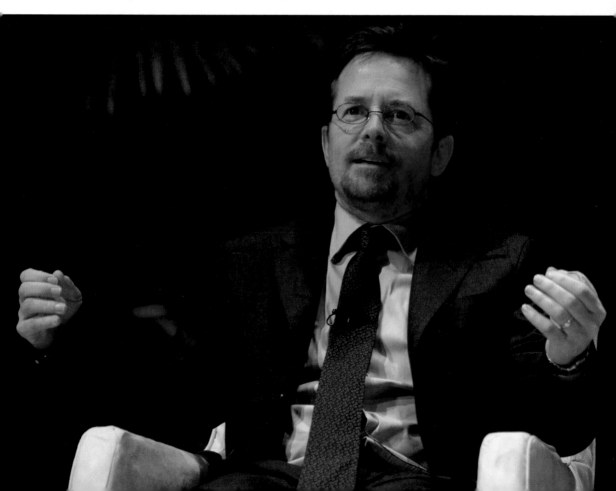

believe the potential for the therapy is enormous—people who suffer from debilitating diseases such as cancer, heart disease, diabetes, Parkinson's disease, Alzheimer's disease, spinal cord injuries, and many other incurable conditions may be able to emerge from their illnesses and go on to live long and healthy lives.

But the use of one form of stem cells, known as embryonic stem cells, requires withdrawing cells from very young embryos, thus destroying them. Many opponents of stem cell research, including some of America's leading conservative political leaders, have opposed embryonic stem cell research. They maintain that destroying embryos means denying opportunities for those embryos to develop into babies. Says Senator Sam Brownback of Kansas, an opponent of embryonic stem cell research, "If an embryo is a life, and I believe strongly that it is life, then no government has the right to sanction their destruction for research purposes."[2] Opponents have also raised alarms that the research could lead to the development of reproductive cloning—the production of a fetus not through the natural act of sexual intercourse but by inducing cells to reproduce in a laboratory dish.

A patient suffering from vascular disease receives an injection of his own stem cells. Doctors hope that the stem cells will rebuild damaged blood vessels and thus improve circulation in the patient's leg and foot.

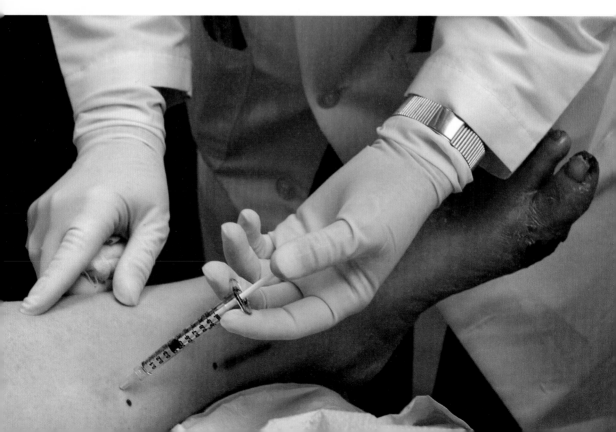

Proponents of embryonic stem cell research counter that the cells are withdrawn from embryos that are no more than a few days old—they are tiny organisms known as blastocysts—and can hardly be regarded as human babies. Moreover, they argue that most embryos employed in stem cell research are donated by in vitro fertilization clinics, where they would have otherwise been discarded. Finally, supporters of stem cell research suggest that by restricting science on cloning, opponents would hinder the development of therapeutic cloning—the use of genetic engineering to cure birth defects, diseases, and disabilities.

Even so, for many years opponents of embryonic stem cell research were able to convince the federal government to withhold virtually all funding for the research. In the meantime, the merits of the research were debated on the floor of Congress, in political campaigns, and in other public forums. Clearly, stem cell research has emerged as a topic that touches many sensitive issues, such as the purpose of science and medicine, the position of the United States as a world leader in technology and science, the ongoing debate that focuses on whether life begins at conception, and whether embryonic stem cell research is, at its core, morally correct.

> "If an embryo is a life, and I believe strongly that it is life, then no government has the right to sanction their destruction for research purposes."[2]
>
> — Senator Sam Brownback of Kansas, an opponent of embryonic stem cell research.

Executive Order

The restrictions on federal funding for embryonic stem cell research ended in March 2009 when President Barack Obama signed an executive order, potentially making billions of dollars available for the research. Obama's order was expected—during the previous year's campaign for the presidency, Obama pledged to end the funding ban. "The majority of Americans from across the political spectrum . . . have come to a consensus that we should pursue this research," Obama insisted. "The potential it offers is great, and with proper guidelines and oversight, the perils can be avoided."[3]

Scientists rejoiced at the news, while political conservatives fumed, indicating that despite the new life Obama breathed into the research, the debate over use of embryos in scientific research is not likely to end soon. Meanwhile, the president's decision will provide researchers with new opportunities to explore the potential of stem cells, giving patients of debilitating diseases hope that cures can be found for their illnesses before it is too late.

Fox predicts that one of the diseases for which stem cells will prove to be particularly effective is Parkinson's. He believes stem cells can be coaxed into becoming dopamine-producing brain cells. He says:

> We know these cells can produce neurons that make dopamine. We also know that dealing with the brain is tricky. You've got to get in there without causing any damage and then figure out how to get the cells to thrive there. It presents a lot of problems, yet embryonic stem cell research is so promising that it's hard to understand the hesitation people have with studying them.[4]

FACTS

- A 2007 Gallup poll found that 64 percent of respondents favor the use of human embryos in scientific research.

- It was formerly believed that Parkinson's disease mostly afflicts people over the age of 60, but in recent years doctors have diagnosed the disease in younger patients, and now up to 10 percent of Parkinson's patients are under the age of 40.

- The embryos discarded by in vitro fertilization clinics are sufficient to meet the needs of all embryonic stem cell research programs in America.

What Are the Origins of the Stem Cell Controversy?

S tudents of Greek mythology are familiar with the story of the Hydra of Lerna, the many-headed water serpent that defeated numerous heroes who believed they could kill the beast by lopping off one or more of its heads. As all those unfortunate heroes were to learn, as soon as they sliced off one head of the Hydra, another would grow quickly in its place.

The story of the Hydra was certainly known to Abraham Trembley, a Swiss naturalist who in 1740 experimented with a tiny animal he found swimming in freshwater ponds. Trembley named the animal "hydra" because its habits mimicked those of its much fiercer mythological version. (Trembley had nothing to fear from this hydra—it is no more than a few millimeters in length.)

When Trembley cut a hydra in two, he noticed its amazing powers to regenerate itself—to grow back the parts he cut off. Moreover, as Trembley examined the critter under his microscope, he noticed that the pieces he cut off grew their own heads and tentacles. "If I had continued to cut them off as they sprouted," Trembley wrote, "no doubt I would have seen others grow. But here is something more than the fable dared invent: the seven heads that I cut from this hydra, after being fed, became perfect animals: if I so chose, I could turn each of them into a hydra."[5]

Trembley's methods of studying the hydra helped establish biology as a science, but he lacked the scientific knowledge to explain why the hydra was able to repair itself. When the answer to that question finally surfaced some two centuries later, it gave birth to the pursuit of stem cell therapy.

The Significance of the Blastocyst

By the 1890s biologists were deep into the study of cells, their structures, and habits. By then they had concluded that cells fall into two classes: somatic cells, which compose all parts of the body—skin, bone, organs, fluids, and other tissue—and germ cells, or gametes, which are cells that enable reproduction to occur. Gametes in the testes produce sperm; ovaries produce eggs.

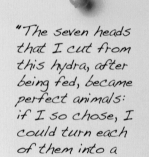

"The seven heads that I cut from this hydra, after being fed, became perfect animals: if I so chose, I could turn each of them into a hydra."[5]

— Abraham Trembley, eighteenth-century Swiss naturalist who pioneered the study of cellular regeneration.

Nearly every animal—including the human—develops after a sperm fertilizes an egg. Together they form a single cell, called a zygote. In the case of a human, over the course of several days the zygote rapidly divides, doubling its size every 12 hours. When the zygote has grown to 150 to 200 cells, or after about 5 days of development, it is called a blastocyst. The blastocyst has not yet developed any features but contains cells that have the potential to develop into every organ that will eventually be present in a human body. In fact, a blastocyst is smaller than a grain of sand. Within a few days the blastocyst travels down the female's fallopian tube and implants in her uterus. At this point the blastocyst is called an embryo, and organ development begins in earnest. After 8 weeks of development, the embryo is referred to as a fetus. The zygote, blastocyst, embryo, and fetus, therefore, all represent different stages of human development.

The stage of development that is important in stem cell research is the blastocyst phase. It is this stage in which the cells are undifferentiated, meaning they have yet to become different, or specialized. In other words, when they are in their undifferentiated stage, cells have not yet become skin cells, blood cells, or brain cells.

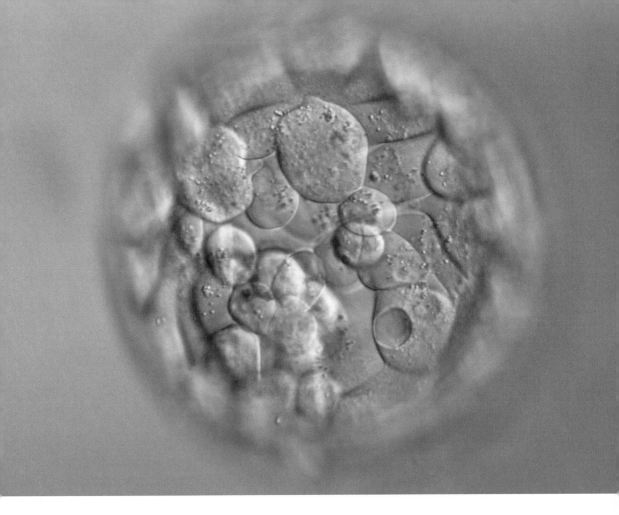

In 1895 a German zoologist, Valentin Häcker, first used the term *stammzelle*—in English, "stem cell"—to describe undifferentiated cells found in a blastocyst he withdrew from a crustacean known as a cyclops, a tiny sea animal similar to a lobster.

Flatworms, Newts, and Zebra Fish

Meanwhile, in Great Britain biologist Thomas Hunt Morgan concentrated on flatworms, finding—like Trembley's hydras—they had amazing powers of regeneration. He once cut a flatworm into 279 pieces and watched as each piece regenerated itself into a new flatworm. Like Trembley, Morgan was not sure why flatworms were able to regenerate themselves, but he suspected that if some animals, such as flatworms and hydras, had the power of regeneration, then science could probably figure out ways that bodies of

A specialized microscope captures an image of the hollow ball of cells known as a blastocyst. The blastocyst contains cells that have the potential to develop into every organ found in the human body.

other animals, including humans, could replace diseased or damaged cells with new, healthy cells. He wrote:

> I should like to discuss . . . the question why certain animals seem to lack the power to replace lost parts; and since man himself belongs to this class, the meaning of the fact is of direct and, perhaps, even of practical importance to us; for if we could determine why man does not replace a lost arm or leg, we might possibly go further and discover how such process could be induced by artificial means.[6]

The Sad Case of Christopher Reeve

Christopher Reeve shot to stardom in the 1970s and 1980s when he portrayed Superman in an enormously popular series of movies based on the comic book character. In 1995, though, Reeve's career came to a crashing halt when he was thrown off a horse, sustaining a debilitating spinal injury. Following his injury, Reeve became an advocate for embryonic stem cell research.

Although a quadriplegic confined to a wheelchair, Reeve made speeches, wrote books, and testified before Congress, imploring lawmakers to free up federal funds for stem cell research, which he was convinced would provide a cure for his condition. "I advocate it because I think scientists should be free to pursue every possible avenue," Reeve said.

Reeve died in 2004, five years before federal funding was authorized for embryonic stem cell research. He fell victim to an infection related to his injury. When President Obama signed an executive order permitting the use of federal funds for stem cell research, he pointed out that Reeve had been instrumental in convincing people of the importance of the research.

Quoted in Alanna Nash, "Christopher Reeve Interview: A Hero Onscreen and Off," *Reader's Digest*, October 2004. www.rd.com.

In the ensuing years the answer that eluded Trembley and Morgan made itself clear to other researchers: Flatworms and hydras could direct huge populations of their own undifferentiated stem cells to regenerative purposes. Other species, including newts and zebra fish, seemed to have even more potent stem cells. When one of those animals sustained an injury, the stem cells headed for the trouble zone—regardless of whether it was a fin, a tale, or an internal organ—to regenerate into a new body part. This research led to the determination that stem cells are pluripotent, meaning they have the potential to become any kind of cell in any part of the body.

400,000 Frozen Blastocysts

The next significant developments in stem cell research occurred more than a half century later. In 1956 a patient who suffered from leukemia—cancer of the bone marrow—received the first bone marrow transplant. (Bone marrow is the soft substance inside bones where most cell formation occurs.) The donor was the patient's identical twin. In 1963 Canadian researchers Earnest A. McCulloch and James E. Till concluded that bone marrow contains stem cells that form new bone marrow when transplanted into a recipient. These stem cells were not formed in a blastocyst but in the bone marrow of the adult donor. Therefore, the regeneration was the work of a second type of stem cell—a so-called adult stem cell.

At first scientists believed bone marrow transplants could be successful only in cases in which the donor and recipient are genetically related, but soon researchers discovered that bone marrow transplants involving unrelated patients and donors could also be accomplished. Clearly, the ability of one person's bone marrow to survive and flourish in another person's body showed how well stem cells could adapt to their new environments.

Meanwhile, a very different type of science was under way. For years women who were unable to conceive children had little choice but to face the unfortunate reality that they would never become biological mothers. There are many reasons for female infertility—hormonal imbalances and injuries to the fallopian tubes are among the most common. In 1968 British scientists Robert

"The list of cell-based diseases that could be eradicated through stem cell treatments encompasses almost anything you can think of."[7]

— Eve Herold, public education manager of the Stem Cell Research Foundation.

Edwards and Barry Bavister pioneered in vitro fertilization (*in vitro* is a Latin term that means "in the glass"). They were able to surgically withdraw an egg from a woman's body and, in a test tube, inject her husband's sperm, completing the act of fertilization that her body was incapable of performing on its own. After the egg is fertilized in vitro, it is returned to the womb, where it then goes through natural growth into a fetus. The breakthrough has provided help for many infertile couples. Today there are more than 350 in vitro fertilization clinics in the United States.

The development of in vitro fertilization would also provide a resource for embryonic stem cell researchers. At the clinics, physicians routinely withdraw many eggs from a woman's body, which are then fertilized in vitro. However, only one fertilized egg is returned to the womb. The others are stored for a time in a frozen state in case the first attempt fails and they are needed for repeat implants. In most cases, though, the excess in vitro embryos are eventually destroyed. These fertilized eggs are in the blastocyst phase of embryonic development. Therefore, researchers have found an enormous reservoir of stem cells available at in vitro fertilization clinics. Experts estimate that some 400,000 blastocysts are sitting frozen in liquid nitrogen in the freezers of American in vitro fertilization clinics. Moreover, most polls have shown that couples who no longer need their embryos are willing to donate them to stem cell research.

In 1998 scientists at the University of Wisconsin withdrew the first stem cells from human embryos that were created at in vitro fertilization clinics. Researchers working with human stem cells confirmed what their predecessors discovered about the hydra, flatworm, newt, and zebra fish: Stem cells possess widespread powers to regenerate cells damaged through disease and can be coaxed into differentiating into specific cells throughout the body. In addition, researchers discovered that if stem cells are withdrawn from embryos, placed in a dish, and fed nutrients, they would—for a time—continue to thrive and even grow and duplicate. This process is known as creating a stem cell line. In 1998 scientists at Johns Hopkins University in Maryland created

"Research on embryonic stem cells raises profound ethical questions, because extracting the stem cell destroys the embryo, and thus destroys its potential for life."[9]

— Former U.S. president George W. Bush.

the first stem cell line in a lab dish. By 2001, 64 lines had been created, providing many of the stem cells employed in the various research projects under way at American laboratories.

Federal Ban Enacted

As researchers learned more and more about stem cells, they saw the potential for huge breakthroughs in medical science. Since many diseases and disabilities lead to a breakdown of cells, it is believed that stem cells could be injected into the bodies of patients and coaxed into forming new cells destroyed by those diseases. Patients with diabetes, cancer, and heart disease are regarded as candidates for stem cell therapy. Also, patients with debilitating conditions caused by diseases of the brain and central nervous system—such as Parkinson's, Alzheimer's, and amyotrophic lateral sclerosis, which is also known as Lou Gehrig's disease—may find cures in stem cell therapy. Stem cells could be deployed to help burn victims who have lost skin. Researchers also believe that stem cells could be used to repair spinal cords in patients who have received injuries that have left them confined to wheelchairs. Says Eve Herold, public education manager of the Clarksville, Maryland–based Stem Cell Research Foundation:

> The list of cell-based diseases that could be eradicated through stem cell treatments encompasses almost anything you can think of, including age-related conditions and the process of aging itself. In fact, if and when stem cell treatments become available to Americans, they could end up extending people's life spans well beyond anything one could have dreamed possible a mere 10 years ago.[7]

But as scientists delved deeper into stem cell research, others started raising concerns about the nature of the research. Since the research involves withdrawing cells from a blastocyst and, therefore, destroying a developing embryo, they questioned whether stem cell research is moral. Indeed, long before the full potential of stem cell therapy was realized, the federal government enacted a ban on the use of federal funds to finance research on human embryos.

The ban has applied to the use of federal funds only; state and local governments as well as private foundations and corporations may fund research on embryos. Also, the ban has had no effect on research involving adult stem cells, since those cells are not removed from blastocysts.

At first Congress enacted a temporary ban on embryonic research soon after the 1973 *Roe v. Wade* decision by the U.S. Supreme Court that made abortion legal. Congress reacted to intense pressure by the antiabortion movement, whose leaders feared that legalizing abortion would lead to unnecessary experimentation on fetuses—that some women would volunteer for abortions simply to receive cash payments from the labs. Eventually, Congress turned the issue over to the U.S. Department of Health and Human Services (HHS) to decide whether to keep the ban in place.

The ban stayed intact for decades, even as the significance of stem cell research became more evident. In 1987 HHS established the Human Fetal Tissue Transplantation Research Panel to assess the importance of research on embryos in the eradication of disease. After studying the science for a year, the panel voted 18-3 to support research on embryos. Nevertheless, HHS secretary Louis Sullivan refused to lift the ban. In 1990 Congress, which was controlled by a Democratic majority, enacted legislation to overturn the HHS ban, but Republican president George H.W. Bush vetoed the bill, leaving the moratorium on federal funding intact.

Defying the Dickey-Wicker Amendment

In 1993 Democratic president Bill Clinton took office and soon instructed the new HHS secretary, Donna Shalala, to lift the ban on funding for stem cell research. At that point the antiabortion rights movement mobilized, flooding the White House and Congress with complaints. Although the National Institutes of Health (NIH) spent the next year writing guidelines and assessing which projects to fund, little federal money was directed to embryonic stem cell research. Responding to pressure from the antiabortion movement, Clinton withdrew his approval for stem cell research funding.

Burning Their Notes

The ban on using federal funds for embryonic stem cell research created many obstacles at university labs and similar institutions where scientists were engaged in this work. For example, machines and instruments bought with federal grants could not be used for stem cell research that was being funded by private resources. The situation evolved to the point where scientists had to leave little notes on equipment, reminding them which machines could be used for which projects.

When President Obama lifted the ban on federal funding in 2009, it meant the instruments and machinery bought with federal grants could be used for the stem cell experiments that had previously been funded entirely with private grants. "One of my colleagues out in California said she was going to have a party and burn the Post-it notes," said Jonathan Moreno, a professor of bioethics at the University of Pennsylvania in Philadelphia.

Quoted in Marie McCullough, "Scientists See Big Impact in Obama Move," *Philadelphia Inquirer*, March 10, 2009, p. A-1.

In 1995 Congress passed an appropriations bill that included an amendment written by Republican representatives Jay Dickey of Arkansas and Roger Wicker of Mississippi prohibiting the use of federal funding for research in which human embryos are destroyed. Clinton signed the bill, but three years later, after the experiments at the University of Wisconsin showed stem cells could be withdrawn from excess blastocysts at in vitro fertilization clinics, he reversed course and authorized the NIH to fund stem cell research. Clinton maintained that the Dickey-Wicker amendment did not apply to embryos stored at in vitro fertilization clinics because the blastocysts "are not a human embryo within the statutory definition."[8] At that point the NIH started accepting grant applications from stem cell researchers.

Clinton opened the door to federal funding for embryonic stem cell research, but it was slammed shut again by early 2001. Soon after taking office in 2001, Republican president George W. Bush ordered the NIH to suspend consideration of the grant applications until he reviewed the policy. On August 9, 2001, in a nationally televised speech, Bush announced his decision: He would sign an executive order authorizing that federal grants could be used to fund research on the 64 stem cell lines that were already in existence, but no new lines could be created using federal assistance. "Research on embryonic stem cells raises profound ethical questions, because extracting the stem cell destroys the embryo, and thus destroys its potential for life," Bush said. "Like a snowflake, each of these embryos is unique, with the unique genetic potential of an individual human being."[9]

For most of the eight years of the Bush administration, Congress remained under Republican control, but stem cell research surfaced as one of those rare issues with support crossing party lines. Moderate Republicans and even some antiabortion Republicans as well as virtually all Democrats in Congress were convinced of the importance of the research. "The scientists know more than the people in the White House," said Senator Arlen Specter, a legislator from Pennsylvania who has battled Hodgkin's lymphoma, a cancer of the lymph nodes. "And the scientists tell us [stem cells] have enormous potential to cure diseases like the one I'm suffering from."[10] In 2006 and 2007 Specter and other proponents of stem cell research in Congress tried to overturn the president's executive order limiting federal funding for embryonic stem cell research. Both times the legislation passed with healthy majorities, but those votes still fell short of the two-thirds majorities Congress would need to override presidential vetoes. "The use of federal dollars to destroy life is something I simply do not support," Bush insisted as he announced his intentions to veto the 2006 bill. "The issue that involves the federal government is whether or not to use taxpayers' money that would end up destroying that life."[11]

"Promoting science isn't just about providing resources. It's about letting scientists . . . do their jobs, free from manipulation or coercion, and listening to what they tell us, even when it's inconvenient."[15]

— President Barack Obama, who signed an executive order in 2009 authorizing the use of federal funds for embryonic stem cell research.

Meanwhile, the 64 stem cell lines approved for federal funding by Bush were becoming exhausted. Indeed, the lines could not continue to replicate stem cells indefinitely, and by 2008 just 21 were still of use to researchers. Also, while research on adult stem cells had continued, it was becoming evident to scientists that embryonic stem cells had much greater powers of differentiation. "There are camps for adult stem cells and embryonic stem cells," says Douglas Melton, codirector of the Stem Cell Institute at Harvard University. "But these camps only exist in the political arena. There is no disagreement among scientists over the need to aggressively pursue both in order to solve important medical problems."[12]

Overturning the Ban

Although many private foundations, biotechnology companies, and even some state governments invested in embryonic stem cell research, it was clear that without the billions of dollars that could be provided by the NIH, stem cell research in the United States would continue to crawl along at a slow pace. Some desperate patients, seeking the therapy they believed could save their lives, made trips to European and Asian countries where stem cell research was actively pursued.

In cities and towns across America, support for embryonic stem cell research was growing. "Why shouldn't [couples who undergo in vitro fertilization] be allowed to donate those embryos to federal research to save lives?" asked Senator Robert Menendez of New Jersey. "We allow people to donate organs to save lives: why couldn't a couple, if they so choose, donate their frozen embryos instead of simply discarding them? We can do this ethically and still cure illnesses, enhance lives, and hopefully even save lives."[13]

A 2008 poll conducted by *Time* magazine found that the majority of Americans agreed with Menendez: 73 percent favored using discarded embryos to conduct stem cell research, while just 19 percent opposed the research, with 8 percent unsure. "America is ready for . . . the federal funding of embryonic stem cell research," insisted Sean Tipton, president of the Coalition for the

Advancement of Medical Research, a Washington, D.C., group that supports stem cell research. "Just as it does with other kinds of promising technological and medical research, the federal government must fund embryonic stem cell research."[14]

As the 2008 presidential campaign got under way, the major party candidates found themselves disagreeing on many issues—how to address the threat of terrorism, how to save the faltering American economy, how to end the war in Iraq—but there was no disagreement between them on the future of embryonic stem cell research. Both major party candidates for president, Democrat Barack Obama and Republican John McCain, said they would overturn Bush's ban on federal funding for stem cell research. Obama was elected, and on March 9, 2009—just a few weeks after entering office—he signed an executive order that cleared the way for federal funding of embryonic stem cell research.

In signing the order, Obama said that stem cell research had been kicked around the political arena for too long, and that it was time to give the science a chance to flourish. He said:

> Promoting science isn't just about providing resources. It's about letting scientists . . . do their jobs, free from manipulation or coercion, and listening to what they tell us, even when it's inconvenient. It is about ensuring that scientific data is never distorted or concealed to serve a political agenda, and that we make scientific decisions based on facts, not ideology.[15]

Even with federal funds now flowing into embryonic stem cell research, it will likely be years if not decades before scientists start showing meaningful results—if, indeed, positive results ever do emerge from the research. In the meantime opponents of the research plan to continue making their case—that it is immoral to destroy embryos, even though the embryos in question may contain just a handful of undifferentiated cells. Therefore, despite Obama's belief that science should be kept apart from the political arena, opponents of stem cell research may find they have no other place in which to make their case.

FACTS

- A 2007 study published in the journal *Science* surveyed 1,000 couples at 9 in vitro fertilization clinics, finding that 60 percent of infertile couples would be willing to donate some or all of their remaining embryos to science.

- Of the 400,000 frozen embryos stored at in vitro fertilization clinics, about 8,000 are destroyed each year.

- Following President George W. Bush's 2001 executive order banning most federal aid for embryonic stem cell research, the National Institutes of Health approved about $1 billion a year in funding for adult stem cell research, but just about $50 million annually for embryonic stem cell research.

- In the years in which the number of viable stem cell lines in the United States dwindled from 64 to 21, more than 100 new lines were created in Asian countries where embryonic stem cell research is supported with government aid.

- A few weeks before Bush vetoed the 2006 legislation to permit funding for stem cell research, a poll released by the Coalition for the Advancement of Medical Research indicated 72 percent of respondents were in favor of the research.

- In 2007, 63 U.S. senators voted to overturn Bush's ban on funding for embryonic stem cell research, but the total fell 3 votes short of the majority needed to override a presidential veto; in the House, 247 representatives voted to overturn the ban, which was 43 votes short of a two-thirds majority.

- President Ronald Reagan was supported throughout his career by antiabortion advocates, but after leaving the White House, he developed Alzheimer's disease and eventually died of complications from the disease. After his death, former first lady Nancy Reagan became an ardent proponent for stem cell research.

CHAPTER TWO

What Benefits Could Stem Cell Research Offer?

Blake Dell'Arriga's parents suspected something was wrong with their son when, at the age of three, he had not yet started talking. At first Blake's parents were told by his doctors not to worry—that speech is often delayed in many toddlers—but at the age of four, Blake started stumbling and having other problems with his coordination.

When he started having seizures, the California boy's parents took him to a neurologist, who diagnosed Blake with Batten's disease, a rare neurological disorder caused by the death of cells in the brain. Eventually, victims undergo personality changes, slow learning, and clumsiness. They also lose their eyesight. There is no known treatment, and most victims die in childhood.

In early 2008 Blake and his stepfather, Jeremy Jaeger, boarded a plane to China, where Blake underwent experimental embryonic stem cell therapy at a hospital in Beijing. Within a short time of Blake receiving injections of stem cells, his parents and doctors noticed positive changes. The boy seemed to have developed better muscle control and coordination; he could hold his head up for longer periods and appeared to be more communicative than before. In other words, his condition was no longer deteriorating, but instead showing slight improvements. "Our world was just rocked when Blake was diagnosed with Batten's disease," said Blake's mother, Dawn. "Now, every second of his life is meaningful to us. Going all the way to China wasn't our first choice, but it was almost our only choice and definitely the right one as

Blake has had clear improvement since he's returned. Every day, he's stronger and stronger than before."[16]

Clearly, stem cell therapy has not resulted in a miracle cure for Batten's disease—Blake's abilities at communication and motor control are still far below those of other children his age. Nevertheless, scientists see great promise in employing stem cells to treat Batten's disease, believing that with experimentation and refinement, children afflicted with the disorder may one day lead normal lives. "There are a lot of scientists who believe [stem cell research is] the most promising area to pursue," said Sean Tipton of the Coalition for the Advancement of Medical Research. "You break your leg and the body can heal the bone. You sever the spinal cord and the body cannot repair that. So there's a great need to find a way to help the body to regenerate nerve cells."[17]

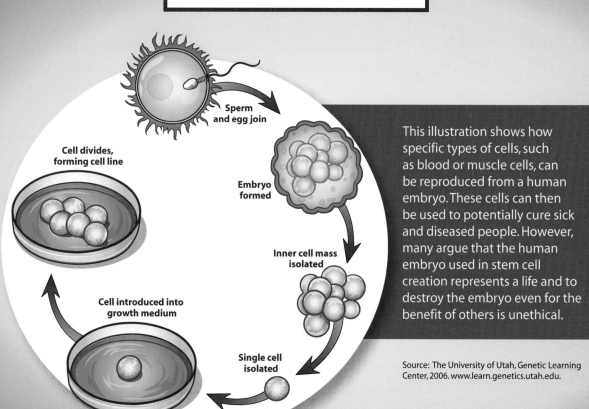

How Stem Cells Are Created

Sperm and egg join

Embryo formed

Cell divides, forming cell line

Inner cell mass isolated

Cell introduced into growth medium

Single cell isolated

This illustration shows how specific types of cells, such as blood or muscle cells, can be reproduced from a human embryo. These cells can then be used to potentially cure sick and diseased people. However, many argue that the human embryo used in stem cell creation represents a life and to destroy the embryo even for the benefit of others is unethical.

Source: The University of Utah, Genetic Learning Center, 2006. www.learn.genetics.utah.edu.

Curative Potential

The curative potential of embryonic stem cells is the main reason many scientists, physicians, and advocates for the ill and disabled have endorsed the research. Stem cells harvested from embryos are expected to offer cures for dozens of diseases that plague millions of Americans. If it is true that embryonic stem cell research has the ability to save and improve lives, it could also save Americans billions of dollars in health-care costs and generate high-paying jobs and lucrative medical industries.

While supporters of the research believe stem cells have great potential, they also caution that the technology is still young. At this point, as with Batten's disease, there are still no quick and effective cures to diabetes, Alzheimer's, Parkinson's, and other horrific diseases. Nor are there likely to be such cures for many years if, in fact, those cures materialize at all. Says science journalist Peter Aldhous, a skeptic of stem cell research: "Scientists, politicians and activists of various persuasions have been making a great deal of some very shaky findings. . . . Many of these findings, including some published in the most prominent scientific journals, have proved extremely difficult to repeat. And if other groups do not get the same results despite many attempts, something is clearly wrong."[18]

Certainly, that has been true in the case of stem cell therapy to treat Batten's disease. While Blake Dell'Arriga has shown some improvement since receiving stem cell injections, other young Batten's disease sufferers have not and have died despite receiving stem cell injections. One young Pennsylvania boy even showed substantial improvement after receiving stem cell therapy at the same Beijing hospital as Blake, but then his condition regressed and he died. "We don't want people to think this is the best thing since sliced bread,"[19] cautioned Robert Steiner, a Batten's disease researcher in Portland, Oregon.

It is clear, though, that due to the long-standing ban on federal funding for most embryonic stem cell research, scientists have been unable to fully explore the potential of the ther-

"You break your leg and the body can heal the bone. You sever the spinal cord and the body cannot repair that. So there's a great need to find a way to help the body to regenerate nerve cells."[17]

— Sean Tipton, president of the Coalition for the Advancement of Medical Research.

Growing a Liver in the Lab

British scientists have taken the first small steps toward growing human organs from stem cells. In 2006 scientists at Newcastle University created an artificial liver, about the size of a coin, in the laboratory by using stem cells drawn from the blood of an umbilical cord. After they were separated from the blood, the stem cells were placed in a machine developed by the National Aeronautics and Space Administration to mimic weightlessness—in a gravity-free environment, stem cells are known to multiply more quickly. Finally, the British scientists injected hormones and chemicals into the cells to coax them into growing into liver tissue.

The liver is regarded as an ideal organ for creation through stem cells because of its ability to regenerate its own tissue. British researchers believe they are at least 15 years away from growing a full-size human liver from stem cells. Nevertheless, they envision the day when they can use a patient's own cells to produce an artificial liver and then provide the organ for a transplant.

apies. For this reason, it remains to be seen if stem cell research could lead to miracle therapies or whether its promise exceeds its capability.

The Pluripotent Promise

Because embryonic stem cells are pluripotent, scientists regard them as biological blank slates with the ability to repair or regenerate new human tissue—in effect, to cure and treat a myriad of diseases. They envision being able to coax stem cells into replacing damaged cells in heart valves, for example, for a patient dying of heart disease. Or they could replace damaged cells in kidneys for someone in dire need of a transplant or provide cells for new bone marrow for someone dying of leukemia.

In fact, some research has indicated stem cells could be coaxed into growing into whole new organs, such as kidneys or livers. No longer would a patient in need of a liver transplant have to wait for one to be harvested from an organ donor—a new liver could be grown out of embryonic stem cells. "Imagine what this research could mean to our returning veterans, coming home with traumatic brain injuries," says Senator Barbara A. Mikulski of Maryland. "There [is] a cornucopia of new opportunities for new breakthroughs."[20]

In addition to curing disease, saving health-care costs, and improving the lives of millions of Americans, embryonic stem cell research is embraced by scientists for its potential to offer insight into organogenesis, the science of how human beings are formed. It also could teach scientists valuable lessons about pathogenesis, or the step-by-step development of disease. Writes the Religious Action Center of Reform Judaism, a supporter of embryonic stem cell research: "American medicine stands on the brink of being able to drastically improve the lives and futures of more than 128 million Americans who currently suffer from debilitating diseases and conditions."[21]

Treatments in China and the Dominican Republic

As the Blake Dell'Arriga case shows, American patients who seek embryonic stem cell therapies have had to go elsewhere to receive the treatment because the federal funding ban in America has limited the availability of such treatments in the United States. The hospital in Beijing where Blake received his treatment, Tiantan Puhua Hospital, has pioneered stem cell therapies in China, and several Americans have sought treatment there as well as in hospitals in other Asian countries and in Europe. In addition to Batten's disease, physicians at Tiantan Puhua have also treated patients suffering from Lou Gehrig's disease, cerebral palsy, traumatic brain injury, stroke, Parkinson's disease, multiple sclerosis, spinal cord injuries, and other debilitations.

Ricci Kilgore did not go to Beijing for her stem cell treatment, but she was still forced to leave the United States. At one time, she was a world-class athlete with hopes of making the U.S. Olympic team in the pole vault competition, but in 2000 her spine was crushed in an automobile accident. The incident left her a paraplegic at the age of 19. Confined to a wheelchair, Kilgore felt only numbness below her waist. Doctors told her she would never walk again.

In 2001, with the federal ban on embryonic stem cell research firmly in place, Kilgore learned about the work of William Rader, an American physician practicing in the Dominican Republic. At a cost of more than $25,000, she received 4 injections of stem cells at Rader's clinic. After the first injection she could stand. After the second she was able to take 100 steps with the aid of a walker. Over the next 7 years, she returned to the Dominican Republic for additional injections. Kilgore is still debilitated and confined mostly to a wheelchair, but she can sometimes walk unassisted and climb stairs, and some feeling has returned to her legs. "This

A French teen paralyzed in a diving accident awaits stem cell injections at China's Tiantan Puhua Hospital in Beijing. The hospital's stem cell treatments for conditions such as stroke, spinal cord injuries, and cerebral palsy have attracted patients from around the world.

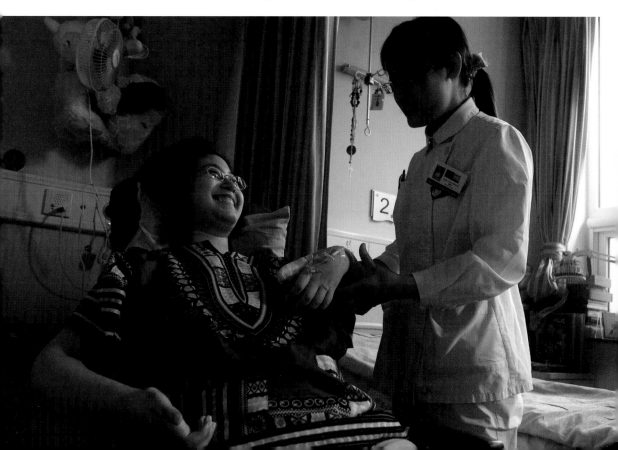

Can Stem Cells Cure Diabetes?

Type 1 diabetes is a disease that attacks cells in the pancreas that produce insulin, a vital chemical that processes sugar in the body, enabling it to be used as fuel. When the body lacks insulin, as it does when a person suffers from diabetes, vital organs can break down. Loss of eyesight is often a typical complication among people who suffer from diabetes. Potentially, diabetes can be fatal.

Actress Mary Tyler Moore is a leading proponent for using stem cell therapy to cure type 1 diabetes. The star of such vintage TV sitcoms as the *Dick Van Dyke Show* and the *Mary Tyler Moore Show*, Moore has suffered from diabetes for 40 years. Retired from acting, she lives quietly in Connecticut. The disease has taken a toll on Moore; today she is nearly blind. "Science is on the verge of many treatments that can and will lead to a cure of this disease," says Moore, "but we can't make that final leap without federal funding to supplement ongoing efforts, especially in the area of stem cell research."

Evidence has surfaced suggesting stem cell research can be successful in treating type 1 diabetes. A 2007 British study of 15 diabetics found their bodies started producing insulin again after receiving stem cell injections.

Quoted in W. Reed Moran, "Mary Tyler Moore Lobbies for Diabetes Research," *USA Today*, July 9, 2001. www.usatoday.com.

wasn't supposed to happen," Kilgore says. "But it did. I can walk. It's amazing."[22]

Kilgore also leads something of an active life. She has moved to Colorado and taken up monoskiing, and she is able to glide down steep mountain slopes on one ski alongside other skiers. She has hopes of making the U.S. Disabled Ski Team and competing in the 2010 Paralympics. She also swims, works out in the gym, and rides horses. "I know that I inspire people with all that I can do, and that's a good thing,"[23] she says.

On the other hand, stem cell treatments have also fallen far short of expectations. The family of Shawna Weil, a 17-year-old Stewartstown, Pennsylvania, high school student, spent $40,000 for stem cell treatments at Tiantan Puhua after she suffered traumatic brain injury in a car accident. The accident left Weil in a near vegetative state. She is minimally conscious, unable to talk, receives nourishment from a feeding tube, and is confined to a wheelchair. Initially, the stem cell injections seemed to be helping, but Weil eventually regressed, and her condition is now no different than it was before she received the treatments at Tiantan Puhua. Still, the Weils do not regret their experience in China and are convinced that stem cell therapy is the best hope for their daughter. "She has no quality of life," says Weil's mother, Lorraine Weil, "so I will constantly search. We've got to do something."[24]

As the Kilgore and Weil cases show, the cost of stem cell treatments can be very expensive. In addition to the fees for the therapy itself, patients and their families must pay for travel, meals, and accommodations for several months in a foreign country. When patients seek therapies outside the United States, they have to bear the cost on their own because private insurance companies in America generally will not pay for experimental therapies conducted in foreign countries. Still, some American families have been willing to shoulder the cost if it means finding cures for horrific diseases.

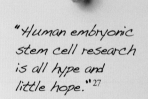

"Human embryonic stem cell research is all hype and little hope."[27]

— Judie Brown, president of the American Life League.

In fact, due to the federal funding ban, there are few embryonic stem cell experiments in America that are in the human trial phase—most research is still conducted on laboratory animals. In many of those cases, the results have been promising, providing evidence that stem cell therapy is more than just theoretical. Scientists can point to actual experiments showing how the health of the subjects improved with stem cell transplants.

In a 2006 experiment at Johns Hopkins University, scientists administered injuries to the spinal cords of 15 lab rats that resulted in paralysis. Those rats were then injected with stem cells. In 11

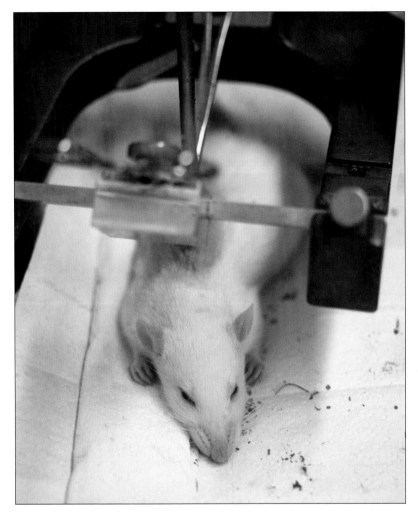

In this photograph, stem cells are harvested from a laboratory rat. Laboratory rats have also been injected with stem cells as part of research into reversing spinal cord injuries and treating various debilitating illnesses.

of the cases, the rats made substantial recoveries, regaining movement in their legs and the ability to walk. In all cases, the stem cells were employed to repair nerve damage in the spinal cords of the rats. "This is proof of the principle that we can recapture what happens in early stages of motor neuron development and use that to repair damaged nervous systems,"[25] said Douglas Kerr, the neurologist who led the Johns Hopkins study.

More Hype than Hope?

But not everyone is convinced of the curative potential of embryonic stem cell research. In fact, whether embryonic stem cells are capable of doing what their supporters claim remains to be seen—

there have been few breakthroughs in medical science attributed to embryonic stem cell research. While this may have been caused, in part, by the severe funding restrictions placed on embryonic stem cell research, it is also due largely to the extreme complexity of the research. Marcus Grompe, a professor of genetics at Oregon Health and Science University, says:

> The truth is that the potential of embryonic stem cells for curing human diseases is unknown. It is therefore factually wrong to state that limitations on embryonic stem cell research are preventing life-saving cures, and it is equally false to claim that embryonic stem cells have no therapeutic potential. At this point, we simply don't know—and without the appropriate research, we will never know.[26]

Because embryonic stem cell research is still a developing field of study, its opponents have called it an overexalted branch of science fiction and doubt that any of what supporters claim is possible will ever be realized. "Human embryonic stem cell research is all hype and little hope,"[27] said Judie Brown, president of the American Life League, which opposes abortion rights as well as embryonic stem cell research. Others suggest there have been significant, even dangerous, complications with embryonic stem cell therapies. In some clinical studies embryonic stem cells have formed tumors after being transplanted in test animals. In one study reported by Israeli researchers, a 13-year-old boy developed cancerous tumors in his spine and brain after receiving stem cell treatments for four years for a rare genetic disorder known as ataxia-telangiectasia. "This doesn't mean the research should be stopped," insisted Ninette Amariglio, the Tel Aviv University cancer specialist who reported the case, "but it should be done in a careful and extensive way."[28]

Moreover, programming stem cells to turn into specific organ cells has also proved to be incredibly challenging and a feat that some doubt can be done. In other words, stem cells dispatched to cure a liver disease or heart defect do not always make it to the targeted organs—they may simply be rejected by the body. In 2008 researchers at Stanford University School of Medicine in

California reported that all laboratory mice injected with human embryonic stem cells had died, meaning that the stem cells were attacked by the immune systems of the mice. "[This result] is not a disappointment, it's more of a reality check," said the lead researcher, radiologist Joseph Wu. "I think there is some promise to [embryonic stem cells], but you don't want to be foolish and say these cells are going to cure things in the next five years."[29]

The type of negative results shown in the Israeli and Stanford University studies have prompted those who oppose using embryos in research to argue that the benefit of stem cell research is at best untested and at worst grossly exaggerated. Says David A. Prentice, a biochemist and research fellow at the antiabortion rights group Family Research Council, "Embryonic stem cells have many hurdles to overcome before they might be useful."[30]

Even those who believe embryonic stem cell research is promising concede that its benefits are likely to be decades away. Says British stem cell expert Robert Winston, "I am not entirely convinced that embryonic stem cells will, in my lifetime, and possibly anybody's lifetime for that matter, be holding quite the promise that we desperately hope they will."[31] On the other hand, researchers who work in this field have confidence that given enough time and the right tools, they can overcome these challenges. Say Elizabeth G. Phimister and Jeffrey M. Drazen, editors of the *New England Journal of Medicine*, "Although these challenges are daunting, none are beyond theoretical reach."[32]

The Promise of Therapeutic Cloning

Some stem cell researchers believe that immune systems will be more likely to accept stem cells if they are genetically similar to the body's existing cells. To accomplish this they are experimenting with a process known as somatic cell nuclear transfer (SCNT). SCNT is also known as therapeutic cloning.

With SCNT, stem cells are not withdrawn from blastocysts donated by in vitro fertilization clinics. Instead, this highly complex technique involves withdrawing the nucleus from a human somatic cell and inserting it into an unfertilized egg that has had its nucleus removed. In humans and other mammals, all cells except gametes are somatic cells. All internal organs, skin, bones, blood, and other tissue are composed of somatic cells, which contain a complete set of the body's DNA.

Therefore, the process essentially injects a complete set of genetic information from the somatic cell—46 chromosomes—into an egg. In natural reproduction, a complete set of genetic information is created when an egg and sperm each bring 23 chromosomes into the union. One way to think about SCNT is to think of the egg as being "impregnated" by the complete genetic information of the somatic cell, rather than pairing up with a sperm to do so. After being infused with the somatic cell, the egg starts to divide, similar to how it would after naturally being penetrated by a sperm. After a few days, a blastocyst will form that is genetically identical to the donor of the somatic cell.

The potential of creating stem cells through therapeutic cloning is believed to be enormous. Since stem cell lines created from SCNT have the advantage of being genetically identical to the donor, researchers think they might be better tolerated by a host's immune system. But their benefit may even go beyond finding cures for diseases—stem cells created through therapeutic cloning could help researchers follow the evolution of diseases, watching them grow from their earliest and simplest forms.

Essentially, researchers think they can learn about disease development and function by studying stem cell lines that are linked directly to particular diseases. For example, if scientists use SCNT technology to take a somatic cell from a person with Alzheimer's disease and inject it into an unfertilized egg, the resulting stem cell line would contain genes that relate directly to Alzheimer's disease. This disease-specific line is believed to give researchers an isolated look at the genetic characteristics of the disease being studied. Therefore, by watching how diseases develop from their most basic forms, researchers hope to find ways to alter human cells genetically so that they would be strong enough to resist the disease when it enters the body.

South Korean scientist Hwang Woo Suk (left) claimed to have cloned a human embryo and extracted stem cells from it. This would have been an important breakthrough in therapeutic cloning, but Hwang later admitted that he faked his research.

Scandal in South Korea

However, researchers have a long way to go before SCNT will directly contribute to human embryonic stem cell research or to curing disease. At this time no human stem cell lines have been derived from SCNT research. In 2005 a South Korean scientist claimed to have accomplished this feat, but his research was later determined to have been fraudulent.

Indeed, the legitimacy of embryonic stem cell research and therapeutic cloning received a setback when Hwang Woo Suk, a top stem cell researcher in South Korea, admitted to faking his work. In 2004 Hwang published the results of research in

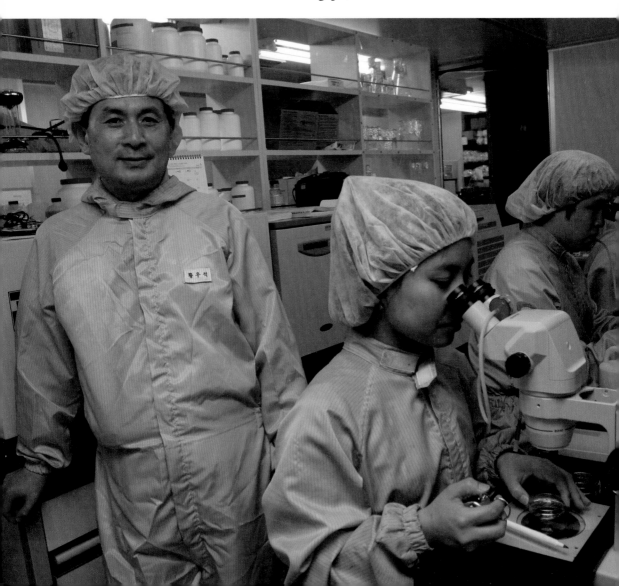

which he claimed to have cloned a human embryo and extracted stem cells from it. If Hwang's achievement had been legitimate, it would have been an important breakthrough in therapeutic cloning. It would have meant that a patient could provide healthy cells from a scraping of skin, which would then produce undifferentiated stem cells that could be returned to the body to repair damaged organs. Hwang said he faked the research because he felt he was under tremendous pressure to show positive results.

During a visit to a South Korean hospital in 2004, Hwang promised a boy crippled in an automobile accident that he would one day walk again. "My son asked him, 'Doctor, can you make me stand up and walk again?'" said the boy's father, Kim Je Eun. "And Dr. Hwang said, 'You will walk again, I promise.'"[33] However, soon after the results of Hwang's work were published, rumors about the legitimacy of the research surfaced in the scientific community. Finally, in November 2005, Hwang admitted that he had fabricated the evidence and was forced to resign from the research institute he headed.

Despite the scandal in South Korea as well as the setbacks suffered in Israel and elsewhere, stem cell researchers push on. Now that federal funding will pour into the coffers of research institutions in America, the research promises to move further into human trials. Says Eve Herold of the Stem Cell Research Foundation:

> [Scientists] must learn how to identify stem cells at every stage of development, as well as how to stimulate differentiation and desired cell types. Then, they need to learn how to keep the cells from over-dividing once they are in the body, to avoid the dangers of tumors and other side effects. Nevertheless, with all the promise already demonstrated in animal experiments and in lab dishes, there is every reason to believe that each of these obstacles will be overcome.[34]

"I am not entirely convinced that embryonic stem cells will, in my lifetime, and possibly anybody's lifetime for that matter, be holding quite the promise that we desperately hope they will."[31]

— Robert Winston, British professor, scientist, and politician.

FACTS

- If only one-quarter of the 400,000 frozen embryos stored at in vitro fertilization clinics are donated to stem cell research, they could be expected to create 2,000 to 3,000 new lines for research.

- Batten's disease is relatively rare; it afflicts 3 out of 100,000 babies born in the United States.

- In 1982 scientists first altered the DNA in embryonic stem cells drawn from mice, giving them the power to engineer the genes that could cause diseases. Not until 2009, though, were scientists able to alter the DNA in stem cells drawn from larger laboratory animals, such as rats.

- Each year about 15,000 people donate organs, about half of whom provide their organs when they die. Even so, about 100,000 Americans are waiting for organ donations.

- Some 5.3 million Americans suffer from Alzheimer's disease, including 2.7 million over the age of 85; by 2031, it is estimated that 3.5 million people over the age of 85 will be afflicted with Alzheimer's disease.

- By the time most people are diagnosed with type 1 diabetes, as many as 80 percent of the insulin-producing cells in their bodies have been wiped out by the disease.

Should Scientific Promise Outweigh Moral Concerns?

Because stem cell research involves the destruction of embryos, it raises many of the same moral issues inherent in the abortion and birth control debates. These moral arguments on stem cell research are born out of opinions about the earliest stages of human development. The central question in the debate is, Can a small group of undifferentiated cells be regarded as human life?

"However small or undeveloped an embryo might be, it is still human," insists David P. Gushee, a professor of Christian ethics at Mercer University in Georgia. "It is what every one of us was at the earliest stage of life—because life develops along an unbroken continuum, from fertilization until natural death."[35]

Many proponents of stem cell research argue, though, that a blastocyst is not human life but, rather, a group of cells that has the *potential* to become human life. "To claim that a fertilized egg within days of conception is a human person is a totally platonic view of the human person," argues Rosemary Radford Ruether, professor of feminist theology at Pacific School of Religion in California. "It means there is a human soul fully present in a tiny speck of germ plasma."[36]

The moral debate over the destruction of the human embryo has raged since the earliest days of stem cell research. Certainly, it has been more than an intellectual duel fought among theologians, philosophers, scientists, and politicians. In 2001, when President George W. Bush suspended most federal funding for embryonic research, it was with the conviction that even a blastocyst possesses a human soul and that he would not authorize the federal government to assist in the destruction of those embryos. Therefore, the moral principles of the president were responsible for sharply curtailing the advancement of embryonic stem cell research for eight years.

Bush's successor, President Obama, has taken a much more secular view of the issue. During the 2008 campaign for the presidency, Obama was asked whether he thought embryos in these very early stages possess human souls. Obama, who has professed to being a deeply religious Christian, answered that he believes it is "above my pay grade"[37] to make that assessment. In other words, it is Obama's belief that it is not within the power of any human being to decide when a soul enters a body. A few months later he signed the authorization that enabled federal support for embryonic stem cell research.

> "However small or undeveloped an embryo might be, it is still human. It is what every one of us was at the earliest stage of life—because life develops along an unbroken continuum, from fertilization until natural death."[35]
>
> — David P. Gushee, professor of Christian ethics at Mercer University.

From Embryo to Infant to Adult

Those who consider stem cell research immoral are appalled by the process, which requires the destruction of the embryo in the blastocyst phase. Some, especially those who are religious, believe that a soul is created at the moment of conception. This is the Catholic Church's position on the origins of life, for example. For Catholics and others the destruction of even the single-celled zygote amounts to the loss of a human soul.

In fact, a 2004 Harris Poll found that a person's level of opposition to embryonic stem cell research is influenced by the degree to which they are religious. Those who describe themselves as "very religious" are much more likely to completely oppose the research (23 percent) than those who describe themselves as "not at all" or "not very" religious (4 percent). Born-again Christians are more likely to oppose stem cell research than other Christians, and Catholics are more likely to oppose it than Protestants.

But many people who do not regard themselves as religious harbor doubts about interrupting the course of human development for the sake of science. They ground their position not in religion, but in the logical evolution of human development: Since a blastocyst will eventually become a fetus—which will eventually become an infant, which will eventually become an adult—they argue that destroying the blastocyst is similar to ending the life of an adult person. Even at the cellular level, they contend, the humanity of an embryo is evidenced by the fact that if the embryo is fertilized in vitro, then frozen and later thawed and implanted in a woman's womb, it would continue its development to birth and beyond.

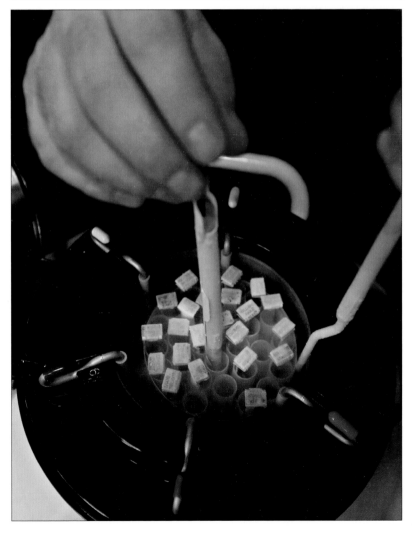

A scientist removes a vial containing frozen human embryos from the liquid nitrogen tank in which it was stored. A thawed embryo implanted in a woman's uterus can lead to a viable pregnancy.

Snowflake Children

President George W. Bush's opposition to the use of discarded embryos from in vitro fertilization clinics for research stemmed from his position that the potential development of the embryos into human beings outweighed the benefits offered by the research. To underscore his point, the president delivered speeches on his opposition to embryonic stem cell research while surrounded by so-called snowflake children—people who have been born via in vitro fertilization after their embryos spent time in a freezer.

In some cases after couples no longer need their embryos to produce their own children, they have been willing to donate their frozen embryos to other couples in which the woman is sterile—unable to produce eggs. In such cases the embryos are thawed and implanted in the new mother's womb, where the fetus grows as though the embryo is her own. "Each of these children began his or her life as a frozen embryo that was created for in vitro fertilization, but remained unused after the fertility treatments were complete," said Bush at a 2006 press conference in the company of several "snowflake" children. "These boys and girls are not spare parts. They remind us of what is lost when embryos are destroyed in the name of research."

Quoted in The White House, "President Discusses Stem Cell Research Policy," July 19, 2006. www. whitehouse.gov.

Robert P. George, a philosophy of law professor at Princeton University in New Jersey and a member of President Bush's Council on Bioethics, makes no distinction between the humanity of an embryo and the humanity of a baby who has been born in a hospital delivery room. "The adult that is you is the same human being who, at an earlier stage of your life, was an adolescent, and before that a child, an infant, a fetus and an embryo," he says. "Even in the embryonic stage, you were a whole, living member of the species *Homo Sapien*."[38] It is for this reason that opponents of stem cell research sometimes refer to the embryo as "a human being in the embryonic stage," "an embryonic human being," or even as "embryonic children." This language helps to underscore their main points: that embryos are people waiting to happen and that the only difference between embryos and people, in their view, are age and size.

"Smaller than a Grain of Sand"

But not everyone agrees that embryos are persons in the full sense of the word. It is morally troubling for some Americans to assign the same rights, characteristics, and liberties to a cluster of 200 undifferentiated cells as to a baby that has limbs, organs, and sensory skills. Indeed, a blastocyst does not have any of the qualities that are normally associated with life, humanity, or personhood—such as the capacity to move, think, feel, or experience. Because of this, supporters of embryonic stem cell research reject the accusation that destroying the blastocyst is tantamount to the murder of a person.

From this perspective embryos at the blastocyst stage are viewed as more of a biological fact with the potential for personhood rather than a person at its earliest age. David Holcberg and Alex Epstein, analysts at the Ayn Rand Institute—a think tank that defends individual rights—are two experts who argue it is inappropriate to put embryos and persons on equal moral and political footing. Explain Holcberg and Epstein:

> Embryos used in embryonic stem cell research are manifestly not human beings—not in any rational sense of the term. These embryos are smaller than a grain of sand, and consist of at most a few hundred undifferentiated cells. They have no body or body parts. They do not see, hear, feel, or think. While they have the *potential* to become human beings—if implanted in a woman's uterus and brought to term—they are nowhere near *actual* human beings.[39]

"These embryos are smaller than a grain of sand, and consist of at most a few hundred undifferentiated cells."[39]

— David Holcberg and Alex Epstein, analysts at the Ayn Rand Institute.

Holcberg, Epstein, and other proponents of stem cell research find the concept of rights completely inapplicable to biological matter that is more "prehuman" than human in the full sense of the word.

One way in which ethicists try to prove that embryos are distinctly different from persons is by examining how society reacts when they are naturally lost—in other words, when women miscarry. Miscarriages are very common, and often a woman miscarries so early in the pregnancy she never even knows she was pregnant. This is why it is estimated that more than 50 percent of all pregnancies end in miscarriages.

But society does not view the loss of an embryo via miscarriage the same way it views the death of a child or even the birth of a stillborn fetus. While such tragic events are usually dealt with by holding a burial, funeral, or similar rite, rarely do those type of proceedings accompany miscarriages, especially ones that occur in the first few days of conception. Says Harvard University philosophy professor Michael J. Sandel, "The way we respond to the natural loss of embryos suggests that we do not regard this event as the moral or religious equivalent of the death of infants."[40]

Given that argument there must be a significant difference between an infant and an embryo, and this is exactly what supporters of embryonic stem cell research maintain. A 2007 poll conducted jointly by ABC News and the *Washington Post* indicates that the majority of Americans agree with this distinction; this is why 61 percent of them support stem cell research that involves destruction of human embryos.

Acorns Are to Oak Trees as Embryos Are to Humans

Even the most ardent supporters of embryonic stem cell research do not deny that there is a connection between a blastocyst and a person—it is a clear biological fact. Ethicists, politicians, and researchers who support stem cell research do not deny this link but argue there is an important moral difference between the two stages of life. Sandel has likened the relationship between embryos and humans to acorns and oak trees. He reasons that although every oak tree got its start from an acorn, oak trees and acorns are themselves very different things. Should an acorn in his front yard get eaten by a squirrel, he would consider it a wholly different kind of event than if a giant oak tree in his yard fell down during a violent storm. "Despite their developmental continuity, acorns and oak trees differ," he says. "So do human embryos and human beings, and in the same way."[41]

Sandel's argument holds that just as acorns are potential trees, human embryos are potential human beings. They are related, but the degrees by which human life develops are too significantly different to be lumped together as one and the same.

Sandel and others who embrace the acorn–oak tree analogy are careful to point out that even though embryos should not be considered full human beings, it does not mean they are to be disrespected. Indeed, there are very few Americans who would stand for the destruction of embryos in order to test a new line of cleaning products or to make advances in elective cosmetic surgery. But it is the very nobleness of stem cell research that, for supporters, makes the destruction of embryos an acceptable loss. For them, the morality of curing disease in potentially millions of people outweighs the gravity of destroying an embryo.

"The way we respond to the natural loss of embryos suggests that we do not regard this event as the moral or religious equivalent of the death of infants." [40]

— Michael J. Sandel, Harvard University philosophy professor.

Priorities of the Living

Supporters of stem cell research believe it is unjust to put the priorities of embryos above the priorities of the already living. They view the protection of embryos from stem cell research as nothing less than sentencing to death the children and adults who are suffering from diseases that could be cured by the research. It is immoral, in their opinion, to protect embryos at the expense of people who suffer from diabetes, Alzheimer's, Parkinson's, Batten's, and other debilitating and ultimately fatal illnesses.

Senator Robert Menendez has accused opponents of stem cell research of "keeping our parents, our children, and our friends locked in wheelchairs and hospital beds. . . . By not allowing embryonic stem cell research, we are prohibiting individuals from pursuing their rights, we are blocking them from a possible cure or treatment, and we are standing in the way of their freedom."[42]

If embryonic stem cell research would truly allow researchers to make astounding new discoveries—such as the ability to create new tissues and organs and to find cures for dozens of diseases—then supporters think it is immoral to block these cures from being found. They view arguments over the rights of embryos as an unnecessary delay that condemns those suffering from disease to pain and early death. "If the 'pro-lifers' ever achieve the ban they seek on embryonic stem cell research," write Holcberg and Epstein, "millions upon millions of human beings, living or yet to be born, might be deprived of healthier, happier, and longer lives. . . . [It is absurd] to force countless human beings to suffer and die for lack of treatments, so that clusters of cells remain untouched."[43]

Several polls, including a 2007 survey by the Pew Research Center for the People & the Press and the Pew Forum on Religion & Public Life, confirm that the majority of Americans feel this way on the issue. The Pew survey, for example, found that when asked which they thought was more important—using stem cell research to find cures, or protecting the potential life of human embryos—51 percent of respondents said that finding cures is more important, while 35 percent said not destroying embryos is more important. (Fourteen percent said they are not sure how they feel.) Pollsters from NBC News and the *Wall Street Journal* asked a similar question and got a stronger set of results. Seventy-one percent of respondents said that using stem cells from human embryos is worth potentially finding cures for diseases such as cancer, Alzheimer's, Parkinson's, and spinal cord injuries, while just 22 percent thought the potential for finding cures for diseases is not worth the destruction of embryos. (Seven percent said they are unsure.)

Experimenting on Humans

But for those who believe that embryos should be accorded similar rights and respect as children and adults, performing medical research on them is immoral and inappropriate. They are primarily opposed to performing life-threatening research on one class of people for the sake of another. "However noble the ultimate pur-

Stem Cells and Eugenics

Many opponents of embryonic stem cell research believe the science could lead to eugenics, the use of genetic engineering to produce perfect specimens of the human race. The notion was first raised in an 1869 book, *Hereditary Genius*, authored by Francis Galton, a cousin of Charles Darwin. While Darwin developed the theory of natural selection—which said that over time (usually millions of years), species developed traits that enabled them to adapt, survive, and flourish—Galton favored using science to give evolution a nudge.

Over the years eugenics was endorsed by prominent intellectuals, but after World War II the idea fell out of favor after it was learned that Nazi scientists conducted genetic experiments on concentration camp inmates. Says Christine Rosen, a fellow of the Ethics & Public Policy Center, a Washington, D.C.–based group that studies the role of religion in public life:

> Embryonic stem cell promoters claim that their science will lead to cures for a range of diseases and the alleviation of much human suffering. And they denounce those who question the ethics of their pursuit as backward or blindly religious. But as we continue to debate the ethics of embryonic stem cell research, it is worth recalling that movements waged in the name of scientific progress often leave a troubled legacy.

Christine Rosen, "Remember Then, Now," *National Review*, March 3, 2005. www.nationalreview.com.

pose for which it is done," says William J. Saunders, a bioethics expert with the Family Research Council, "we have always agreed it is wrong to kill one human being to benefit another."[44]

Saunders and others go so far as to claim that stem cell research is a violation of the Nuremberg Code, which was adopted after World War II. The code was developed in response to inhumane experiments conducted by the Nazis on their prisoners, including sterilizing adults, dissecting live infants, and injecting deadly chemicals into people to see how their bodies would react.

Since the adoption of the Nuremberg Code, the international community has roundly condemned research that exploits, experiments on, or threatens the lives of one group of people for the sake of helping another group. People who view embryos as people regard stem cell research in the same vein. The Nuremberg Code states, in part, that if human subjects are to be used in experiments, researchers must obtain their voluntary consents. Obviously, an embryo is incapable of giving consent, providing opponents with ammunition to argue that embryonic stem cell research violates the code. Furthermore, the Nuremberg Code prohibits an experiment from being conducted if there is the potential for the subject of the experiment to become disabled or killed as a result of it.

On this point, too, opponents see a violation, as the harvesting of stem cells destroys the embryo. Says Christian ethics professor David P. Gushee: "They are exploited, or experimented on, or harvested—choose whatever term you like—by some members of the human community for the benefit of others. They die that others might (someday maybe) find healing for their maladies."[45] And Judie Brown of the American Life League urges Americans to consider that "even if killing human embryonic children produced miraculous cures, it is always immoral to pursue the research."[46]

Yet supporters of embryonic stem cell research raise another aspect of the Nuremberg Code to defend it—that which requires all experimentation to serve the greater good of society. Certainly, they argue, there are few pursuits greater for society than finding cures to diseases afflicting millions of men, women, and children. Furthermore, supporters point out that medical advances from a single embryo could benefit millions of people down the line. Because they do not view the embryo as a human being, sacrificing the embryo to save so many, in their minds, is worth it.

Troubling Science

By using the process of somatic cell nuclear transfer (SCNT), or therapeutic cloning, the blastocyst is not destroyed. Still, opponents of stem cell research find it difficult to accept therapeutic cloning as an acceptable alternative.

Opponents argue that in therapeutic cloning, the human reproductive act has been replicated in a laboratory through the use of test tubes, needles, and petri dishes. Scientists counter, though, that the researchers are not performing reproductive cloning—they are not creating human life in a petri dish with the express purpose of growing a child from cloned cells. Rather, they are engaged in therapeutic cloning: taking healthy cells, cloning copies, and then using the healthy cells for a therapeutic purpose—to eradicate disease. Says Richard Furlanetto, scientific director of the Juvenile Diabetes Research Foundation, "Stem cells have the unique capacity to become any type of cell, tissue or organ as they mature, yet they cannot themselves develop into a full human being."[47]

And yet, opponents argue that therapeutic cloning should not even be tried. They argue that the relationship of embryonic stem cell research to cloning could lead to troubling science, particularly the prospect that SCNT might lead to reproductive cloning—the process of actually creating life in a lab dish. Reproductive cloning was most famously accomplished by scientists in Scotland who cloned a sheep named Dolly in 1996. Many critics believe it is impossible to prevent reproductive cloning while legalizing and encouraging therapeutic cloning. Some biologists and ethicists repeatedly point out that although the two are discussed as if they are separate and unrelated procedures, reproductive and therapeutic cloning are both forms of cloning—the only difference is what happens to the cells that are cloned. Says Saunders: "Cloning is often discussed as if there were two different kinds of cloning [but] all successful cloning is reproductive. That is, once cloning results in a living single-cell human being, reproduction, by definition, has occurred. It does not matter for what purpose this cloning was accomplished—another member of the human species exists."[48]

Saunders and others worry that allowing cloning for even research purposes will bring on an onslaught of problems that

> "By not allowing embryonic stem cell research, we are prohibiting individuals from pursuing their rights, we are blocking them from a possible cure or treatment, and we are standing in the way of their freedom."[42]
>
> — Senator Robert Menendez of New Jersey.

Therapeutic Cloning May Cure Parkinson's Disease

Researchers have been able to cure Parkinson's disease in mice by creating cells through somatic cell nuclear transfer (SCNT), which is also known as therapeutic cloning. In 2008 a team of scientists at Memorial Sloan-Kettering Cancer Center in New York cloned cells from the tail skin of laboratory mice, then injected them into the brains of the mice. The cloned stem cells developed into neurons that released dopamine. The cognitive abilities of the mice that received the cloned stem cells improved after they received the implants.

Researchers said the cells worked well in the mice because the mice donated the cells to themselves—therefore, the cloned cells were genetic matches. When cloned cells were injected from donor mice into other mice, the cells died and the Parkinson's symptoms in the recipients did not improve. "It demonstrated what we suspected all along, that genetically matched tissue works better," says Viviane Tabar, a member of the Memorial Sloan-Kettering research team.

Quoted in Maggie Fox, "Cloned Mice Cells Treat Parkinson's," ABC Science, March 24, 2008. www.abc.net.au.

society is not prepared to face, such as the creation of embryo farms that produce cloned babies. Indeed, the very notion of cloning raises complex political, religious, moral, and human rights questions about how to classify life that is not unique and produced through the sexual act by biological parents. Therefore, most people who object to the use of SCNT in stem cell research do so on the grounds that cloning is too dangerous a technology to use for stem cell research, even if it would herald benefits.

But supporters of SCNT say the technique could yield such amazing discoveries it is worth pursuing and could be safeguarded by adopting just a few guidelines that would ensure its responsible use. These would include a formal ban on reproductive cloning, passing laws that remove incentives for women to sell their eggs to researchers for money, and requiring that cloned embryos be frozen and their growth stalled before the point at which their development complicates the ethics surrounding their use.

Culture of Life or Culture of Death?

Both sides of the stem cell research debate claim to support a "culture of life" and accuse their opponents of supporting a "culture of death." Opponents of stem cell research view the destruction of embryos as murder, whereby potential humans, who have no voice of their own, are sacrificed so that other humans may benefit. Their desire to protect embryos from experimentation and destruction is to them part of a pro-life platform that they would like to see upheld throughout America. As Saunders has asked: "Would any of us wish to live in a society where one class of human beings is manufactured to suit the preferences of others? What, indeed, will it mean to be 'human' in such a society?"[49]

Yet from the other side's perspective, people who stand in the way of stem cell research are the ones fostering a culture of death—the death of thousands of men, women, and children who suffer and die in the absence of cures that embryonic stem cell research could provide. From this perspective those who oppose stem cell research based on their goal of protecting the sanctity of life have missed the point of the argument. Denying cures, and thus life, to millions under the banner of a pro-life position seems incongruent. As Alex Epstein suggests, "To uphold [the opposition of stem cell research] in the name of the sanctity of life is a colossal fraud."[50] With both sides claiming to represent the true culture of life, it is clear that the morality of embryonic stem cell research will continue to be debated by a polarized American public for many years to come.

"However noble the ultimate purpose for which it is done, we have always agreed it is wrong to kill one human being to benefit another."[44]

— William J. Saunders, bioethics expert with the Family Research Council.

FACTS

- About 53 percent of Americans think it is immoral to use human cloning technology to develop cures for disease, according to a study by the Virginia Commonwealth University Life Sciences Survey.

- In July 2000 Pope John Paul II declared embryonic stem cell research and cloning among the "evils of Western culture."

- By 2005 fewer than 100 children had been born from embryos that were at one time frozen at in vitro fertilization clinics.

- About 2 percent of couples who conceive through in vitro fertilization request that their excess frozen embryos be donated to other couples for procreation—the others either authorize the clinics to discard the embryos or make them available for scientific research.

- Animals were first born through reproductive cloning in the 1950s, when scientists split the nuclei in frog embryos to create tadpoles. Since then fish, sheep, and cows have been born following reproductive cloning. To anyone's knowledge a human child has never been created through reproductive cloning.

- In 1996 Dolly the sheep was cloned from a single cell drawn from the udder of a six-year-old ewe.

Are There Effective Alternatives to Embryonic Stem Cell Research?

S tem cells are not found only in new human embryos. They are also present in bone marrow, brain matter, skin, intestines, teeth, organs, and other places in the body. These stem cells are known as adult stem cells, and since they can be extracted from a child or adult without causing the destruction of an embryo, research into adult stem cells is vigorously endorsed by opponents of embryonic stem cell research.

In fact, many experts who support embryonic stem cell research believe adult stem cells may also serve the same purpose as embryonic stem cells. They, too, can be coaxed into replicating cells damaged through disease or injury, potentially providing cures for such diseases as Alzheimer's, Parkinson's, and diabetes.

But that does not mean researchers are willing to drop investigation of embryonic stem cell therapies. Proponents of stem cell research contend that both types of stem cells must be studied. "We don't know at this point which will be better for what," says Stanford University stem cell researcher Helen Blau. "We need to learn from both. We need to learn the differences, the relative advantages, and we learn a tremendous amount by comparing the two cells."[51]

The Safest Option

Like embryonic stem cells, adult stem cells are undifferentiated. They are found among other cells in the body, and their purpose is to replace cells that become damaged either through disease or injury. There are places in the various tissues, organs, and fluids of the body known as stem cell niches, which is where the adult stem cells reside, often for many years. Adult stem cells remain dormant until they are needed.

A form of adult stem cell is also found in the blood of the umbilical cord, the tube of tissue with which a mother supplies nutrients to her fetus, as well as the placenta, the bag of thin tissue that surrounds the fetus in the womb. Typically, cord blood is withdrawn from the placentas and cords donated by mothers after

Stem cells can be harvested from blood found in the umbilical cord and placenta (pictured). After a woman gives birth, blood from both can be frozen until it is needed for stem cell harvest.

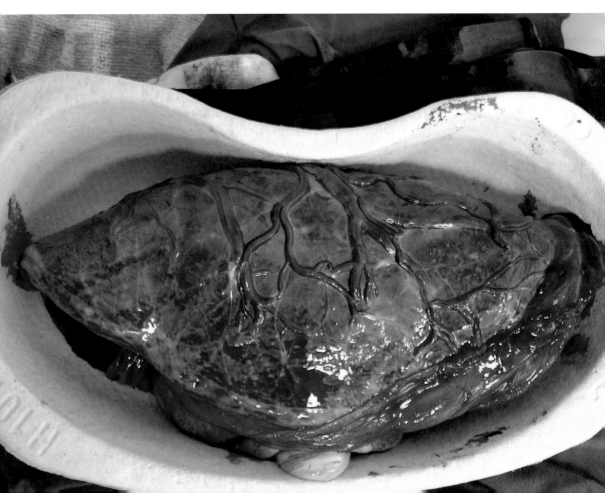

they give birth. The blood is then frozen until it is needed for stem cell harvest. These stem cells are often called cord blood cells.

As with embryonic stem cells, adult stem cells are pluripotent. While stem cells found in the brain, for example, do a very good job of differentiating into brain cells when they are needed due to a head injury, research has also found that undifferentiated adult stem cells drawn from brain matter can evolve into cells that can be used to repair other organs. Says Wolfgang Lillge, a physician and science journalist:

> It has been known for about 30 years that stem cells are present in the tissue of the adult, but it was assumed that they could only form cells of a particular tissue. That is, reprogramming them was considered impossible. In recent years, however, pluripotent stem cells were discovered in various human tissues—in the spinal cord, in the brain, in the . . . various organs, and in the blood of the umbilical cord. These pluripotent stem cells are capable of forming several cell types—principally blood, muscle, and nerve cells. It has been possible to recognize, select, and develop them to the point that they form mature cell types.[52]

"The greatest advantage of adult stem cells is that it's usually possible to use a person's own stem cells, which is the safest stem cell option for people."[53]

— Jean Peduzzi-Nelson, professor of anatomy and cell biology at Wayne State University School of Medicine in Michigan.

Another advantage of adult stem cells is that in many cases the patient can be his or her own donor, meaning that there is virtually no chance the body's immune system will reject the cells. "The greatest advantage of adult stem cells is that it's usually possible to use a person's own stem cells, which is the safest stem cell option for people," says Jean Peduzzi-Nelson, professor of anatomy and cell biology at Wayne State University School of Medicine in Michigan. "This avoids the problems of rejection, disease transmission, chromosomal abnormalities and uncontrolled growth,"[53] which can lead to tumors.

While adult stem cells may have some distinct advantages over embryonic stem cells, many scientists believe there are also disadvantages in using adult stem cells. When researchers examine cells in an organ or in tissue, they are able to find relatively few undifferentiated adult stem cells among the massive amount of cells under study. Therefore, adult stem cells are often difficult to find.

Moreover, the pluripotency of adult stem cells is believed to be limited—although they can be coaxed into differentiation, they lack the widespread ability of embryonic stem cells to be fashioned into all manner of other uses. And once the adult stem cells have been withdrawn from the body, researchers have found it much more difficult to grow stem cell lines from them. In other words, they are not believed to be as long-lasting or as pliable as embryonic stem cells. According to a publication of the National Institutes of Health, "Adult stem cells are often present only in minute quantities, are difficult to isolate and purify, and their numbers may decrease with age."[54]

Hope for Heart Patients

There is, of course, one tremendous and undeniable difference between treatments involving adult stem cells and those involving embryonic stem cells: To date, treatments employing adult stem cells have cured diseases or otherwise improved the quality of life of patients, while therapies involving embryonic stem cells have largely not. Soon after the first bone marrow transplants more than five decades ago, scientists concluded that it was the adult stem cells in the donor's marrow that replaced the cancer-stricken cells of the recipient. Says Wesley J. Smith, a consultant to the California-based Center for Bioethics and Culture, which opposes embryonic stem cell research:

While there have certainly been successes in embryonic stem cell experiments in animal studies—many of them hyped to the hilt in mainstream media reports—the numbers pale in comparison with the many research advances

Adult Stem Cells May Cure AIDS

In Germany adult stem cell therapy was used successfully to treat a man suffering from human immunodeficiency virus (HIV), the virus that often leads to the fatal disease AIDS. The patient sought stem cell therapy to treat leukemia, but doctors believed the therapy could also be effective in controlling the man's HIV. As the donor of the adult stem cells, which were drawn from bone marrow, they selected a person whose blood contains a mutation of a gene that is found to be particularly resilient against HIV. After receiving the stem cell transplant, the patient appeared to have no trace of HIV in his blood.

Doctors cautioned that the therapy is still highly experimental and even dangerous. Doctors must intentionally destroy the patient's immune system before introducing the new stem cells, which establish a new immune system. In the meantime, the patient is very vulnerable to infections that could prove fatal. Nevertheless, doctors hope that in time, the therapy can be employed on a widespread basis. Said Gero Hutter, the German physician who performed the surgery, "For HIV patients, this report is an important flicker of hope."

Quoted in Jacquelyne Froeber, "Man Appears Free of HIV After Stem Cell Transplant," CNN, February 11, 2009. www.cnn.com.

being made with adult and umbilical cord blood stem cells, which are already being used in human patients. . . .

Embryonic stem cells have not treated a single human patient, and only time can tell whether they ever will. Highlighting the progress of adult-umbilical cord blood stem cells—an uncontroversial therapeutic approach that does not require the destruction of human embryos—is a legitimate part of the public discourse.[55]

In the decades since the first bone marrow transplants, stem cells extracted from bone marrow have been transplanted into the hearts of patients, where they have been effective in repairing damaged heart tissue. Many of the patients treated with stem cells had experienced heart attacks or suffered from congestive heart failure, a weakening of the heart that makes the organ incapable of pumping enough blood to meet the body's needs. For many people congestive heart failure can be a fatal condition, but adult stem cells have been effective in bolstering the heart and making it stronger.

Such research is still in its trial phases—by 2006 just 400 heart patients worldwide received stem cells as part of their therapies. And yet the research has shown promising results. A 2004 University of Pittsburgh study focused on 20 heart patients who received coronary bypass operations. (In a coronary bypass operation, a surgeon transplants an artery from another part of the body to the heart, where it is used to carry blood to the rest of the body that would otherwise be blocked by arteries that have become clogged by disease.) During the surgeries 10 of the patients received injections of adult stem cells into their hearts, while 10 received only the bypass surgeries. Six months after the surgeries, the hearts of the patients who received the stem cells were stronger and able to pump more blood than the patients who received the bypass surgeries only. Said Amit Patel, a physician who participated in the study, "We don't know if this [improvement] was due to the growth of new heart muscle cells resulting from the stem cell injections or whether the stem cells coaxed existing cells to come out of hibernation. What we do know is that stem cell transplantation led to significant improvement in cardiac function in these patients undergoing off-pump bypass surgery."[56]

In Franklinton, Louisiana, Aaron Cathcart's congestive heart failure had grown so acute that doctors gave him less than a year to live. Cathcart's heart was so weak that he had to stay indoors whenever the weather dropped below 50°F (10°C)—his heart was too weak to pump enough blood to warm his body in

"When you put the [stem] cells in your spinal cord, they're yours, it's natural, you've got an environment which is a very friendly one, and so the cells will grow."[60]

— Carlos Lima, Portuguese neurologist who has injected adult stem cells into paralyzed patients.

Where Adult Stem Cells Are Found in Humans

Researchers once thought that adult stem cells were only found in bone marrow and a few other select areas of the body. In recent years, however, they have learned that stem cells are found throughout the body, and are far more plentiful than what was originally thought. The following illustration shows other areas where adult stem cells are found.

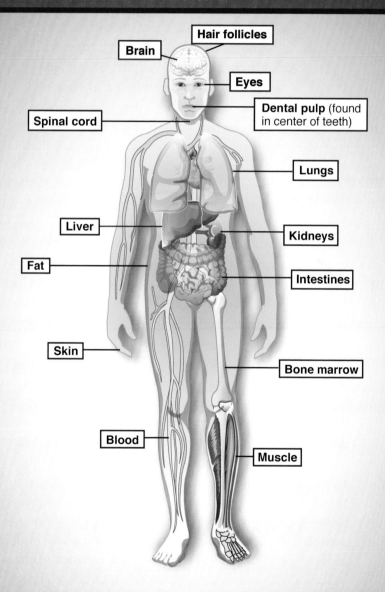

Brain
Hair follicles
Eyes
Dental pulp (found in center of teeth)
Spinal cord
Lungs
Liver
Kidneys
Fat
Intestines
Skin
Bone marrow
Blood
Muscle

Sources: Christopher Thomas Scott, *Stem Cell Now*, p. 66; The National Academies, "Understanding Stem Cells," October 2006. http://dels.nas.edu; Michael Fumento, "Adult Approaches: Will Embryonic Stem Cell Promise Ever Pay Off?" *The American Spectator*, May 2007. www.fumento.com.

cool temperatures. Moreover, he could not walk more than a few hundred feet without collapsing in pain.

With just a few months to live, Cathcart was accepted into an experimental stem cell trial program. A few weeks before Cathcart's surgery, doctors withdrew his bone marrow, harvested the stem cells, and placed them in an incubator so they would multiply. During the surgery his chest was opened and the stem cells were injected into portions of his heart that had been damaged by the disease. Cathcart's recovery was swift and remarkable—within a few months his heart improved and was nearly as strong as a normal heart. "We'd been living with the idea that he only had so long to live; that's not a life you want to live," says Cathcart's wife, Betty. "I was so afraid he might not survive that when [the doctor] came out and [said] everything had gone well, I just fell into his arms. I was just bawling my eyes out."[57] Adds Aaron Cathcart: "People hear 'stem cells' and they think 'killing babies.' People are not distinguishing between the two. These were my own stem cells they used. . . . Everybody has them, and if you increase them in concentration, they can repair your body much better than normal."[58]

> *"The answers are not just going to come from the adult stem cells and it would be extremely short-sighted to shift completely to just adult stem cells."*[62]
>
> — Stanford University stem cell researcher Helen Blau.

Learning to Walk Again

Elsewhere, adult stem cell therapies have been employed for a variety of diseases. At a Louisiana research institution, doctors have treated patients suffering from lower limb ischemia by injecting them with stem cells drawn from bone marrow. Lower limb ischemia is a painful and inflammatory condition caused by the breakdown of veins in the legs; the stem cells helped repair the veins, improving the flow of blood. "The similarity in the recovery of our patients is promising," said Gabriel Lasala, head of TCA Cellular Therapy, which developed the ischemia treatment. "We find that the stem cells, once re-injected, go about forming new blood vessels, thus increasing circulation dramatically."[59] And in Portugal neurologist Carlos Lima has injected adult stem cells into the spinal cords of paralyzed people and has found substantial improvement in their abilities to regain the use of their arms and legs. Says Lima:

I am asking the patient to treat himself, because your own body will know which are the best cells to multiply, how much and in what direction they should go. And the stem cells that we have, our own body has, that's their job. What we are exploiting is the natural role, their instinct to replace and to repair, because nature made stem cells for that.

When you put the cells in your spinal cord, they're yours, it's natural, you've got an environment which is a very friendly one, and so the cells will grow. We ask the cells to do their job, with the cues that come from the environment and from the damaged area. We know that the stem cells will stay active for months, even years. So we hope to get more function even years after the surgery. So what we say to patients is that if you keep improving, even little by little, who knows where you can go.[60]

One of Lima's patients, Laura Dominguez, was injured in a car accident, which paralyzed her from the neck down. She spent two years in a wheelchair, then traveled to Portugal for the stem cell therapy. A year after returning home to San Diego, California, she regained some use of her arms and legs and is learning to walk again. "The first time [I stood] it took, like, three or four people to help me stand up, just to make sure I wouldn't fall," says Dominguez. "I was pretty wobbly. A month ago, I could only stand up a few times and I was really tired. I was beat. And today, I stand up 30 times, 10 seconds each time. And now when I stand I stand on my toes."[61]

Unknown Dangers of Adult Stem Cells

Stem cells drawn from cord blood have also been used effectively, mostly for patients who suffer from anemia, a lack of red blood cells causing severe fatigue, as well as from leukemia and other blood cancers. In all, patients suffering from some 70 diseases have been treated with stem cells drawn from cord blood. As with all stem cell therapies, though, the research is still in experimental phases—by 2006 only about 6,000 patients worldwide had been treated with cord blood cells.

Bone marrow, which appears in this scanning electron micrograph as red spongy material, is rich in stem cells. Stem cells extracted from bone marrow have helped to repair damaged heart tissue, veins, blood vessels, and spinal cords.

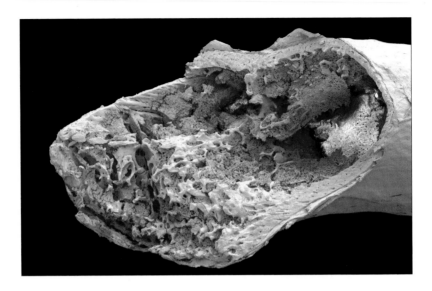

Such success stories are welcomed by advocates of embryonic stem cell research, but they insist that even as adult stem cells are employed to cure disease and improve lives, research into embryonic stem cells must continue. "I feel very strongly we need embryonic stem cells," says Stanford University stem cell researcher Helen Blau. "The answers are not just going to come from the adult stem cells and it would be extremely short-sighted to shift completely to just adult stem cells."[62]

Blau and other scientists also point out that even though adult stem cells have undergone research for some five decades, much is still unknown about them. For example, adult stem cells certainly carry the DNA of the donor, who is often the patient. If adult stem cells are used to treat a patient's cancer, and the cancer is ingrained in the patient's DNA, would the stem cells simply reinforce the patient's cancer? Brain surgeon and cancer researcher Alfredo Quiñones-Hinojosa of Johns Hopkins University is convinced that transmission of cancer through adult stem cells is a very real danger. "We are just beginning to understand this link between stem cells and cancer," he says. "We have to prove that brain cancer stem cells exist. But I think the potential here is real."[63]

Overwhelming Support

And yet there is no question that support for adult stem cell research is overwhelming among people who oppose embryonic stem cell research. Since no embryos are destroyed in adult stem cell research, none of the questions of morality are raised by the research. "The root of the debate really comes down to the ethical question of what's the moral status of a human embryo," says David Prentice, founder of Do No Harm: The Coalition of Americans for Research Ethics, which opposes embryonic stem cell research. "Is it a person or is it a piece of property? And obviously we have no consensus of that in this country."[64]

Opponents of embryonic stem cell research point out that President Obama may have acted hastily in lifting the ban on funding for the research, because in the months before he acted, some new breakthroughs in adult stem cell research had been reported. In late 2007 separate research teams in Japan and at the University of Wisconsin and Harvard University reported that they were able to improve the pluripotency of stem cells drawn from adult skin samples so that that the cells would differentiate as well as embryonic stem cells. These stem cells are known as induced pluripotent stem cells, or iPS cells. Said Bernadine Healy, a physician and medical columnist for *U.S. News & World Report*:

"Embryo-derived cells will remain the gold standard for a while." [68]

— Bernadine Healy, a physician and medical columnist for *U.S. News & World Report*.

> The new creations look and behave like embryonic stem cells taken from seven-day-old embryos; both are able to turn into any type of cell in the body—skin, heart, liver, nerve, you name it. Even better, iPS cells' DNA matches that of the person who provides the skin, which is crucial if the cells are to be used to replace that person's own destroyed or damaged tissue. To date, intense efforts in the United States and around the world to make such genetically matched stem cells through cloning, an alternative approach, have failed miserably.[65]

Given that breakthrough and others, critics of embryonic stem cell research suggest there is no need to destroy human embryos when research on adult stem cells has proved so promising. They also insist that Obama would have done well to maintain the ban at least until the therapeutic value of iPS cells became clearer.

"Wouldn't the humane policy be to fund that line of research?"[66] asks Thomas G. Bohlin, a Catholic priest and vicar of the conservative Catholic organization Opus Dei.

No Moral Triumph

Still, proponents of embryonic stem cell research point out that the iPS cell breakthrough is a relatively recent development and that effective therapies based on the science are probably years away—if, indeed, therapies can ever be developed from that line of research at all. Delaying research into embryonic stem cells until the promise of iPS cells becomes clearer could set embryonic stem cell study programs back years. Since such programs have already been delayed by years due to the funding ban, proponents of embryonic stem cell research contend that it would be foolish to delay the research further.

Indeed, proponents of embryonic stem cell research point out that one of the major hurdles that the research into iPS cells has to overcome is how to rid those cells of viruses, which were injected into the cells to coax them into becoming more pluripotent. A drawback of using viruses is that there is always a danger the viruses could mutate into cancer. "One of the next big milestones will be making these cells without the use of viruses—leaving the cells in a genetically pristine state,"[67] says George Daley, one of the Harvard researchers. A team of scientists at Scripps Research Institute in San Diego, California, may have accomplished this feat, although their work was limited to mice. Results of their research appeared in an online scientific journal in April 2009. The team said it had turned fully formed fibroblast cells—precursors to skin cells—into primitive embryonic-like stem cells without using dangerous genes or viruses.

Experts said this work represents a huge step forward, but more work remains before it can be tried in humans. At this point, Daley says, the iPS cells remain research tools and not agents for therapy. Adds Healy, "Embryo-derived cells will remain the gold standard for a while."[68]

Proponents of embryonic stem cell research insist that pursuing just one path places limitations on a science that is still in its infancy. Healy says there is no need for adult stem cell research to compete against embryonic stem cell research as though the two sciences are rivals in a beauty contest. If, in fact, adult stem cell research eventually proves to be the more effective therapy, she says, proponents of the therapy should not feel as though they have triumphed in a great moral debate; rather, the winners will be the patients of debilitating diseases and injuries whose recoveries can be speeded with the new therapies. "If stem cells can be made better, cheaper, and faster from skin than from embryos," she says, "that's no cause for hand-wringing. It would be a stem cell victory like no other."[69]

FACTS

- **A poll by Virginia Commonwealth University found that 22 percent of respondents believe embryonic stem cell research holds the greatest promise for new therapies, while 17 percent of respondents believe adult stem cell research holds the greatest promise.**

- **A study performed in Ecuador on patients who suffer from congestive heart failure found that their hearts' abilities to pump blood improved by 41 percent within a month of receiving injections of stem cells drawn from aborted fetuses.**

- **The handful of adult stem cells withdrawn from the body must be grown into a massive amount of cells in order for the therapy to be effective; typically, a patient needs an injection of as many as 50 million adult stem cells.**

- **A Chicago study found that 167 angina patients who received adult stem cell injections were able to exercise about a minute longer than angina patients who had not received the injections. Angina is a disease of the heart that often causes weariness.**

- **A Scottish research team has used adult stem cells to repair torn cartilage in knees; such injuries are common among athletes, often resulting in abrupt ends to their careers.**

Should the Government Support Stem Cell Research?

I f embryonic stem cell therapy has the potential to save millions of lives and billions of dollars in health-care costs, should the government help pay for research to develop this therapy? Stem cell research is very expensive. Some states, private biotechnology companies, and foundations have been willing to fund research projects. But because stem cell research is still in its infancy and a return on investments is far from guaranteed, many large drug companies have been hesitant to undertake their own research projects.

Therefore, virtually the only institution that can afford to finance the expensive scientists, lab space, equipment, and other materials needed for the research is the federal government. Whether the U.S. government should fund this research, however, has been a topic of much debate.

New Guidelines Issued

During President George W. Bush's 8 years in office, the federal government agreed to provide limited funding for research on the 64 stem cell lines created prior to Bush taking office in 2001. Bush believed that destroying embryos is immoral, but since the lines had already been created, he found no reason to curtail research that had already started. As for using federal money to create new lines and, therefore, destroy additional embryos, Bush was firmly against it. "We should not use public money to support the further destruction of life,"[70] Bush declared in 2001 as he enacted the 8-year funding ban.

The federal government's position on funding embryonic stem cell research changed in March 2009, when President Obama announced that he would rescind Bush's moratorium on spending. A month later the National Institutes of Health (NIH) issued draft guidelines that would permit funding for stem cell research on embryos that would otherwise be discarded by in vitro fertilization clinics. Officials at the NIH predicted the new guidelines would

In March 2009, President Barack Obama signs an executive order lifting the ban on federal funding for embryonic stem cell research. A month later the National Institutes of Health issued guidelines for research on embryos from in vitro fertilization clinics.

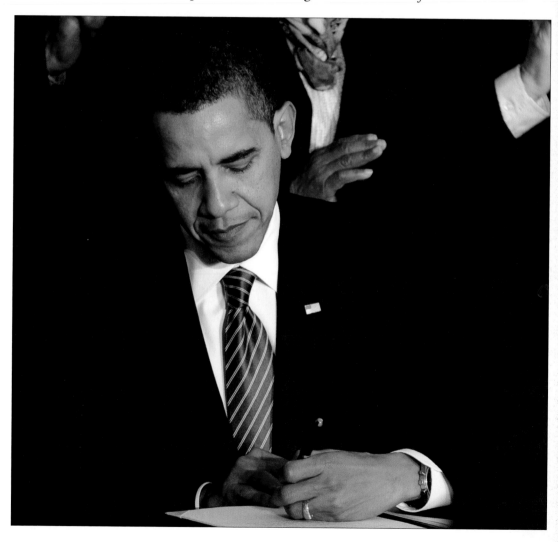

First Embryonic Stem Cell Test Approved

On January 22, 2009, the U.S. Food and Drug Administration (FDA) granted approval to Geron Corporation to perform the first embryonic stem cell test using human subjects in the United States. Geron intends to inject 10 paralyzed people with embryonic stem cells to see whether they regain use of their arms and legs in the therapy. Although the stem cells used in the test were generated by the lines that existed prior to 2001, no federal money had been granted to Geron to develop the experimental therapy it planned to test. Geron pursued the research on its own, using its own resources.

Still, the timing of the announcement certainly showed the new direction planned for embryonic stem cell research in American society. The FDA granted approval to Geron just two days after President Obama was inaugurated, prompting many observers to suggest that the agency had to wait until the Bush administration left office before it could approve an embryonic stem cell test on humans. "It's a milestone and a breakthrough for the field," insisted Ed Baetge, chief scientific officer for a rival biotechnology firm that is also seeking FDA approval for its own human trials.

Quoted in Malcolm Ritter, "First Embryonic Stem Cell Study Approved by FDA," *Huffington Post*, January 23, 2009. www.huffingtonpost.com.

lead to the immediate creation of at least 700 new embryonic stem cell lines. Moreover, the NIH said it had received $10 billion from the Obama administration to fund new scientific research programs in 2009, and it is likely that embryonic stem cell research would receive a large portion of that appropriation.

Still, many members of the scientific community were disappointed by the guidelines, believing they did not rescind all of the Bush administration's restrictions. While there is no question the guidelines would greatly expand embryonic stem cell research in the United States, the NIH's draft rules continued to maintain a ban on funding projects that explore therapeutic cloning—creating stem cells in a laboratory dish specifically for research purposes. Proponents of therapeutic cloning charged that in banning funding for the research, the Obama administration sought to reach a political compromise with conservatives who believe therapeutic cloning—creating cells for specific purposes, such as to mimic disease cells—is immoral. Opponents of cloning believe such techniques give scientists too much control over the creation of life. "I am really, really startled," said Susan L. Solomon, chief executive of the New York Stem Cell Foundation. "This seems to be a political calculus when what we want in this country is a scientific research calculus."[71]

NIH officials defended the guidelines, claiming they were based mostly on the language contained in the legislation drafted by Congress in 2006 and 2007 that sought to overturn Bush's ban. Said Raynard Kington, acting director of the NIH:

> We believe there is broad support to use federal funds to conduct human embryonic stem cell research on cell lines derived from embryos created for reproductive purposes and no longer needed for that purpose. Twice there has been legislation that would allow such use that passed both the House and the Senate. There is not significant broad support for using federal funds for stem cells derived for other purposes.[72]

NIH officials added that in the coming years, it is also possible for the guidelines to be liberalized to permit the use of federal dollars for therapeutic cloning if the public's attitude becomes more accepting of the science and if the science of cloning proves to be of more value. "They did not choose to write guidelines for hypothetical research," insisted R. Alta Charo, a bioethicist at the University of Wisconsin. "They wrote guidelines for the research that is going on and needs to go on. It's a very pragmatic solution."[73]

The public has consistently supported the use of federal funds for embryonic stem cell research. In the years leading up to President Obama's decision to overturn the funding ban, many polls conducted by news organizations showed the American public in support of easing federal restrictions. A 2007 poll conducted by *USA Today* and the Gallup Organization found that 64 percent of Americans believe the president should expand federal funding for embryonic stem cell research, while 31 percent do not. Polls also indicate that the public is growing weary of restrictions entirely: This same poll found that 22 percent of Americans believe no restrictions should be put on the funding of stem cell research, compared with 11 percent who took that position in 2005.

Are Current Stem Cell Lines Adequate?

Though polls show that opponents of federal funding are in the minority, they still represent a sizable number of people who believe that stem cell research is not a business the U.S. government should be backing. Some fear that the proposed rules will gradually become even less restrictive than they appear to be now. "This is clearly part of an incremental strategy to desensitize the public to the concept of killing human embryos for research purposes,"[74] Douglas Johnson of the National Right to Life Committee told the *New York Times*.

Many opponents of federal funding continue to argue that the older stem cell lines are more than adequate for current research needs. They point to evidence showing that many international scientists use samples from those pre-2001 lines for their research. These researchers, they point out, could have obtained access to stem cell lines created in other countries, but they chose to use the American-made lines because they believed them to be of higher quality. What is more, those international research programs were certainly not eligible for financial assistance from the federal government because the United States generally does not fund scientific research projects based in other countries.

One 2006 comprehensive study of all international stem cell research found that just 14 percent of published stem cell research papers were based on cell lines that were not approved by the U.S. government. "The lines are used, in other words, because they are useful,"[75] explains conservative columnist Eric Cohen, who has praised the Bush administration's approach to stem cell research funding as a balance between scientific advances and the protection of nascent human life.

Yet some scientists say that the pre-2001 stem cell lines can be tricky to work with for several reasons. Although more than 700 shipments of stem cells have been sent out to scientists all over the world, many more scientists are interested in doing research. But getting samples takes patience, time, and a lot of money. In fact, scientists complain that samples from these lines are very expensive and formerly arrived with Material Transfer Agreements, contracts that limit what the researchers could do with them. Furthermore, the pre-2001 lines tend to be intolerant of antibiotics, which makes them difficult to work with under some conditions. They also have long "doubling times"—the time it takes for cells to divide—which slows down the pace of research. And, of course, the lines have dwindled in number over the years because they are growing older and losing their ability to produce new cells.

Some experts also complain that the pre-2001 stem cell lines have been contaminated with so-called mouse feeder cells. When stem cell lines are replicated, they are grown on layers of cells drawn from laboratory mice that provide a surface on which the stem cells can adhere and also feed nutrients to the stem cells, keeping them alive over time. The technique was first developed in 1981 and has remained the standard. But scientists worry that the use of mouse cells has tainted the existing stem cell lines, passing along rodent viruses or provoking immune responses from the cells.

Scientists such as Tom Okarma, chief executive officer of the California-based stem cell research company Geron Corporation, claim that mouse feeder cells can be removed from stem cell lines if the researchers are talented enough. "The stuff you hear published that all of those lines are irrevocably contaminated with mouse materials and could never be used in people—hogwash," he says. "If you know how to grow them, they're fine."[76] However, many other scientists have publicly complained about the presence of mouse-feeder-cell contamination and have even given up federal funding of their work to pursue research on stem cell lines grown without the use of mouse feeder cells.

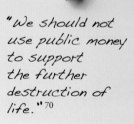

"We should not use public money to support the further destruction of life."[70]

— Former U.S. president George W. Bush.

Does the United States Risk Falling Behind Other Nations?

Supporters of embryonic stem cell research have been warning that U.S. restrictions on funding were leading to a loss of scientists to other countries; unregulated research undertaken by private, possibly "rogue" firms and unethical governments; and jeopardizing the health of Americans who suffer from diseases. Some people even argued that the United States would not be able to maintain its status as a world leader in science and medicine if it did not back a more comprehensive stem cell research program.

A 2006 study published in the journal *Nature Biotechnology* reported that American scientists may be losing their stem cell research lead to scientists from other countries. The study found that non-U.S. scientists published 40 papers on stem cell research in 2004, twice the number published by Americans scientists. Research papers often serve as a good indication for the interest in a particular field of scientific study because they are published at the conclusion of the research. If more research papers are published in a particular field, it shows a high interest by scientists in pursuing research in that field. The papers also offer a valuable resource to other scientists, who may use them to clarify their own research problems or build on the results published by the authors.

Said Jennifer McCormick and Jason Owen-Smith, authors of the *Nature Biotechnology* study: "The U.S. is falling behind in the international race to make fundamental discoveries in [human embryonic stem] cell-related fields. . . . If such discoveries can be translated into therapeutic and commercial opportunities, publication disparities may place U.S. corporations and, more importantly, patients at a disadvantage."[77] In other words, if the United States slips too far behind other countries, it risks the health of its citizens and the money that could be earned from medical discoveries.

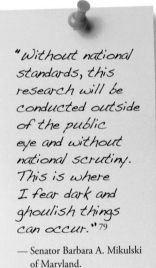

"Without national standards, this research will be conducted outside of the public eye and without national scrutiny. This is where I fear dark and ghoulish things can occur."[79]

— Senator Barbara A. Mikulski of Maryland.

Keeping Stem Cell Research in the Sunshine

There are some indications that American scientists are still leading the way in embryonic stem cell research—but they are doing it in oth-

Economy Hits Stem Cell Research Hard

The dismal economy of 2009 hit embryonic stem cell research hard, as private and public sources for the funding dried up. In 2009 the Maryland state legislature knocked $3 million out of Governor Martin O'Malley's request for $15 million to fund embryonic stem cell research in the state. Meanwhile, in New Jersey, Governor Jon Corzine eliminated $34 million from his state's budget that had been earmarked for embryonic stem cell research.

Corzine's budget cut essentially eliminated all money for the research in 2009. "It's very bad timing to lose this funding right now," said Martin Grumet, director of the Stem Cell Research Center at Rutgers University in New Jersey. "If someone doesn't step up soon to restore it, we're going to lose whatever advantage and momentum we've had compared to places like Australia, England, and Israel that are moving very rapidly."[1]

Actually, though, the poor economy has hit researchers in some of those places, too. In Glasgow, Scotland, clinical trials for a stem cell therapy project for stroke victims at Southern General Hospital have been endangered due to the difficulty in raising the $1.5 million to conduct the trials. "We are struggling all the time to raise money and what we'd really like is some kind of assistance for the 'national good' to see this work continue," said John Sinden, the chief researcher on the project. "We don't want to start this trial and not be able to finish it."[2]

1. Quoted in Adrienne Lu, "Budget Cuts Endanger Stem Cell Research in New Jersey," *Philadelphia Inquirer*, March 4, 2009. www.philly.com.
2. Quoted in Rob Owens, "Stem Cell: Funding Cuts Will Hit Patients," *Sky News*, April 7, 2009. http://news.sky.com.

er countries. Over the last few years, many researchers were attracted to foreign institutes that put few restrictions on both the funding and quality of their research, allowing researchers to make more useful scientific gains in shorter amounts of time. Senator Barbara Mikulski has made this point repeatedly in Congress, and it remains a concern for those who favor the new federal stance. Mikulski has appealed to her colleagues' sense of patriotism in arguing that U.S.-backed stem cell research keeps the nation's best and brightest scientists where they belong—at home. "Our country is sitting back while other countries are moving forward," she has warned. "Scientists are going to other countries to do this research— China, Singapore, Australia, Germany. We are losing our intellectual capital. We are losing young scientists who are choosing other paths because of [American] restraints."[78] At a time when American schools and industries are already struggling to keep up with other countries in math and science, Mikulski and others argue that the United States cannot afford a "brain drain" that would cause it to lose stem cell researchers to other countries.

The lifting of federal funding restrictions has been seen as important for another reason—to ensure that the industry is not driven underground, where it becomes hidden from public scrutiny and oversight. Proponents of stem cell research argue that overly tight restrictions on researchers lead them to seek out funding from other sources and in other nations—places which may have little or no regard for the deep bioethical issues involved in this field. These other sources and nations may not be sensitive to the moral implications of performing research on human embryos and take it past the point that the majority of people agree is reasonable or ethical. For these reasons, Mikulski has said that stem cell research must be kept "in the sunshine," arguing that national standards such as those being proposed are essential for ensuring the research is conducted using state-of-the-art techniques by legitimate university and private labs, employing the top scientists in the field who adhere to the moral and ethical standards adopted by the American Medical Association and other professional groups. "Without national standards, this research will be conducted outside of the public eye and without national scrutiny," says Mikulski. "This is where I fear dark and ghoulish things can occur."[79]

The End of Stem Cell Tourism?

With a new emphasis on stem cell research and development of effective therapies in America, it is believed that Americans suffer-

"They've literally carved him out a new future. He talks. He feeds himself. He laughs. He has a personality again. His cognitive functions have improved dramatically."[80]

— John Brower, whose son has severe brain damage, was treated with stem cells in the Dominican Republic.

ing from debilitating diseases will now seek treatments at home rather than in foreign countries where stem cell therapies have been more available. During the 8 years of the Bush administration, a sort of "stem cell tourism" industry was established as desperate Americans were driven abroad toward more available stem cell technology that promised cures for them and their loved ones. Many American patients have traveled to countries such as China, India, Mexico, the Dominican Republic, and the Ukraine, paying between $12,000 and $50,000 for stem cell therapies that are not

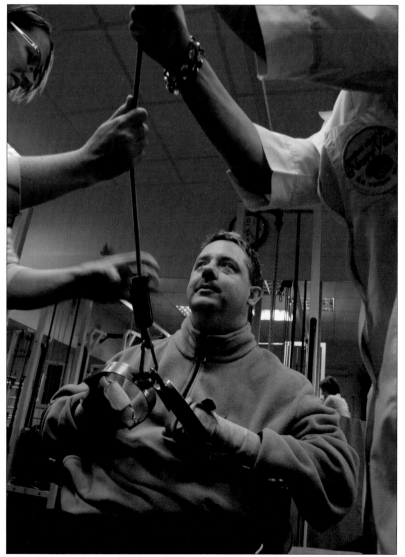

A Michigan man who lost the use of his arms and legs as a result of a car accident undergoes stem cell treatments in a Moscow clinic in 2008. The Bush administration ban on federal funding for embryonic stem cell research led many Americans to seek treatments abroad.

available in the United States. One clinic in China, for example, claims to have treated more than 2,000 patients since 2005, with an 85 percent improvement rate for spinal cord injuries, autism, cerebral palsy, blindness, and other conditions.

John Brower went abroad to seek therapy for his five-year-old son, Jake. After developing a fungal infection in his brain, Jake suffered multiple strokes that left him severely brain damaged, paralyzed, and unable to speak. His doctors said there was nothing that could be done and recommended discontinuing his medical treatment. But Brower mortgaged his home to take his son to the Dominican Republic, where a clinic injected him with human fetal stem cells. After five treatments Brower claims to have noticed an incredible improvement: "They've literally carved him out a new future. He talks. He feeds himself. He laughs. He has a personality again. His cognitive functions have improved dramatically."[80] Brower says that he never would have taken such drastic measures had the same level of care been available in the United States.

But miracle cures in foreign countries have several dark sides that are troubling to American doctors, patients, and policy makers. Says Bernard Siegel, executive director of the Genetics Policy Institute, a Florida group that supports stem cell research: "What if the lab that's doing the procedure won't tell you what cells are being used and is charging $50,000 for an injection, is that fair? Should we condemn this as a scientific community? Should we seek to shut it down?"[81]

Critics also point out that many of the techniques practiced in foreign countries have been developed without clinical testing or government oversight to keep them safe. It is very possible that patients could be further harmed—or even die—as a result of receiving untested experimental therapies in Third World clinics. In fact, American ophthalmologists have questioned stem cell therapies employed at an eye institute in India, which has used stem cell injections to repair damaged corneas in blind people. A 2007 report published by the *Archives of Ophthalmology* warned that the techniques used by the institute can potentially induce "disease transmission through contamination with bacteria, viruses and other infectious agents."[82] Added Ivan Schwab, lead author of the study and

"I absolutely believe that if the federal government messes things up, states have a right to straighten it out."[84]

— Mike Reynolds, an Oklahoma state legislator, who has authored legislation making it a crime to pursue research on embryonic stem cells in Oklahoma.

professor of ophthalmology at the University of California–Davis: "It is a slowly ticking time bomb. I am not saying this work should not be done, on the contrary—but society must be careful with this technology."[83] For all of these reasons, supporters of U.S.-based stem cell research believe it is important to keep research—and the resulting techniques—above board and in American hands.

States May Lead

In the years in which federal support for most embryonic stem cell research was unavailable, some state legislatures provided funding for the research. Since they lack the financial resources of the federal government, their aid was usually delivered in millions rather than billions of dollars. This was not the case in California, where in 2004 lawmakers committed $3 billion over 10 years to fund embryonic stem cell research, provided that a portion of the profits earned from the therapies developed in the state would return to California taxpayers. Other states that have contributed funds to stem cell research include Connecticut, Illinois, Indiana, Maryland, Massachusetts, New Jersey, New York, Washington, and Wisconsin.

On the other hand, some state legislatures have reacted harshly to President Obama's decision to approve federal funding for embryonic stem cell research. Controlled by conservative majorities, these legislatures have moved quickly to ban the use of state money for the research, and some have even made it a crime for scientists to pursue embryonic stem cell research within their borders. About two dozen states that have proposed or enacted such bans include Texas, Oklahoma, South Dakota, Louisiana, and Arizona. "I absolutely believe that if the federal government messes things up, states have a right to straighten it out,"[84] insists Mike Reynolds, an Oklahoma state legislator, who introduced a bill making it a crime for scientists to pursue embryonic stem cell research in his state.

End of Horrific Diseases

Even with the changes now under way, it is likely to take several years if not decades for effective therapies to be developed and instituted on a widespread basis. But proponents insist that the wait is worth it. They point out that medical science has wiped out some of the most horrific diseases known to humans. Over the past century or so, scientists have all but eliminated plagues and influenza pandemics that have wiped out tens of thousands of victims. Polio and tuberculosis—formerly crippling and often fatal diseases—have been largely removed as public health threats from

State Policies on Embryonic Research

Following the 1973 *Roe v. Wade* decision that legalized abortion, many states as well as the federal government took steps to outlaw scientific research on embryos, fearing that some women would undergo abortions for money so they could sell their embryos to laboratories. Those fears have largely gone unrealized, but following President Barack Obama's decision in 2009 to grant federal funding to embryonic stem cell research, some conservative state legislatures have either adopted or proposed bans on the research, making it a crime for scientists to pursue embryonic stem cell research within their borders.

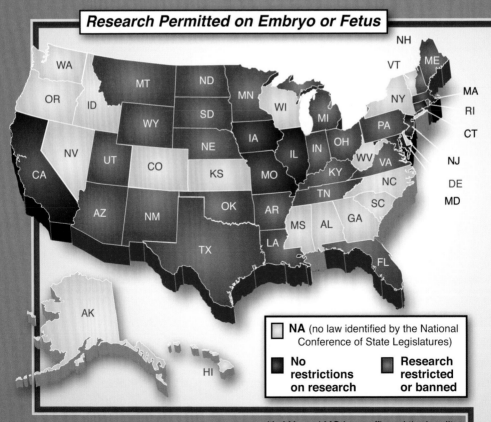

Research Permitted on Embryo or Fetus

NA (no law identified by the National Conference of State Legislatures)

No restrictions on research

Research restricted or banned

IA, MA, and MO have affirmed the legality of embryonic stem cell research but do not offer state funding.

Source: National Conference of State Legislatures, "Stem Cell Research," January 2008. www.ncsl.org.

many corners of the planet. In these cases, it took many years of testing and refining the drugs and therapies that were found to be most effective in treating those diseases. That is why proponents of embryonic stem cell research counsel people to be patient, and that is why they also believe that once paralyzed people start walking again, diabetes patients retain their eyesight, and Alzheimer's patients retain their memories, the moral questions about the research will seem far less significant than they do today.

FACTS

- Although President Barack Obama lifted the federal funding ban on embryonic stem cell research in March 2009, it will still be up to Congress to decide how much money to appropriate to the research. Versions of funding bills were expected to be introduced in both houses of Congress in 2009.

- Only 21 of the 50 new organizations devoted to embryonic stem cell research were started in the United States in 2004, while 29 were launched in other countries, according to a 2006 study published in *Nature Biotechnology*.

- A 2006 study of all international stem cell research found that just 14 percent of published stem cell research projects were based on cell lines not approved by the U.S. government.

- In 2006 the Jülich Research Center in Germany found that Israel publishes the most stem cell research papers per capita, producing 113 papers for every 1 million of its citizens. The United States was ranked sixth, producing 47 papers per million citizens.

- Legislation that would have banned embryonic stem cell research in Georgia was tabled after Representative Amos Amerson, the chair of the House Science and Technology Committee, said the bill would hurt the state economically by driving lucrative scientific research to other states.

Related Organizations

American Life League

PO Box 1350
Stafford, VA 22555
phone: (540) 659-4171
fax: (540) 659-2586
e-mail: info@all.org
Web site: www.all.org

The American Life League opposes abortion rights. By following the "Bioethics" link on the organization's Web site, students can read essays by officials of the league who oppose cloning and embryonic stem cell research.

Beijing Tiantan Puhua Hospital

Tiantan Puhua Stem Cell Treatment Center
12 Tiantan Nanli
Beijing, 100050
People's Republic of China
phone: 86-10-67035566
fax: 86-10-67061799
Web site: www.stemcellspuhua.com

Many Americans undergo stem cell therapies at the Beijing hospital. Visitors to the hospital's Web site can read about the treatments and recoveries of patients who suffer from Parkinson's disease, cerebral palsy, brain trauma, Batten's disease, stroke, and other diseases and debilitations.

California Institute for Regenerative Medicine

210 King St.
San Francisco, CA 94107

phone: (415) 396-9100
fax: (415) 396-9141
e-mail: info@cirm.ca.gov
Web site: www.cirm.ca.gov

The agency was established to distribute $3 billion in state funds to universities, medical institutions, and private laboratories in California that pursue embryonic stem cell research. By following the "All Funded Grants" link on the agency's Web site, visitors can read descriptions about each project that has received funding from the agency.

Center for Bioethics and Culture

130 Market Pl., No. 146
San Ramon, CA 94583
Web site: www.cbc-network.org

The Center for Bioethics and Culture supports embryonic stem cell research and provides information programs to help explain the complicated issues involved in the research. Visitors to the organization's Web site can find essays about stem cell research and download news articles and other materials about stem cell research, cloning, eugenics, and similar issues.

Coalition for the Advancement of Medical Research

2021 K St. NW, Suite 305
Washington, DC 20006
phone: (202) 725-0339
e-mail: CAMResearch@yahoo.com
Web site: www.camradvocacy.org

The coalition is composed of more than 100 universities, medical research institutes, patients' groups, and other advocacy organizations that support embryonic stem cell research. Visitors to the group's Web site can read news stories about scientific breakthroughs, the results of polling on the issue, and the status of legislation by state and federal lawmakers to fund embryonic stem cell research.

Do No Harm: The Coalition of Americans for Research Ethics

1100 H St. NW, Suite 700
Washington, DC 20005

phone: (202) 347-6840
fax: (202) 347-6849
Web site: www.stemcellresearch.org

The coalition has compiled many resources supporting its position that viable alternatives to embryonic stem cell research are available. Students who visit the group's Web site can find news articles on adult stem cells as well as induced pluripotent stem cells, download government reports by the Bush administration's President's Council on Bioethics, and read transcripts of testimony by experts who testified about adult stem cell research before Congress.

Family Research Council

801 G St. NW
Washington, DC 20001
phone: (202) 393-2100
fax: (202) 393-2134
Web site: www.frc.org

By following the "Human Life & Bioethics" link on the council's Web site, students can read a number of essays in opposition to embryonic stem cell research, many written by William J. Saunders, an attorney and expert on bioethics, and David Prentice, a biochemist and research fellow. Students can also view videos promoting adult stem cell research and download a glossary of terms associated with cloning and stem cells.

Gallup Organization

502 Carnegie Center, No. 300
Princeton, NJ 08540
phone: (609) 924-9600
Web site: www.gallup.com

The independent polling institute has conducted many surveys over the years gauging the attitude of Americans toward embryonic stem cell research. By entering "stem cell" into the Web site's search engine, students can find the results and analyses of the institute's polling on the issue.

Genetics Policy Institute

11924 Forest Hill Blvd., Suite 22
Wellington, FL 33414-6258
phone: (888) 238-1423
fax: (561) 791-3889
Web site: www.genpol.org

The institute promotes stem cell research and sponsors the annual World Stem Cell Summit, which features speeches by experts as well as panel discussions that endorse expanding the research. Visitors to the organization's Web site can read news updates on research achievements and follow the efforts of advocates to expand the research. The organization also presents awards to leading stem cell advocates and makes their biographies and stories available on its Web site.

Harvard University Stem Cell Institute

42 Church St.
Cambridge, MA 02138
phone: (617) 496-4050
e-mail: hsci@harvard.edu
Web site: www.hsci.harvard.edu

The Harvard University Stem Cell Institute explores cutting-edge stem cell science. By following the Web site's links to "Public & Press," students can find an overview of stem cell science; copies of *Stem Cell Lines*, the institute's newsletter; and a list of frequently asked questions about stem cell research.

National Institutes of Health

9000 Rockville Pike
Bethesda, MD 20892
phone: (301) 496-4000
e-mail: NIHinfo@od.nih.gov
Web site: www.nih.gov

The National Institutes of Health is the federal government's chief funding arm for medical research projects. The agency will set standards for embryonic stem cell research and decide which projects to fund. Students can find an explanation of the science behind stem cell research by accessing the agency's Web site at http://stemcells.nih.gov/index.asp.

New York Stem Cell Foundation

163 Amsterdam Ave., Box 309
New York, NY 10023
phone: (212) 787-4111
e-mail: info@nyscf.org
Web site: www.nyscf.org

The foundation raises funds for stem cell research projects and also provides numerous public information programs, including conferences and symposiums on the research, staged in New York City. Visitors to the foundation's Web site can learn about stem cell research by accessing the link to "Stem Cells 101." Also, visitors can download copies of the foundation's newsletter, which contains many news stories and updates on developments in stem cell research.

For Further Research

Books

Michael Bellomo, *The Stem Cell Divide: The Facts, the Fiction, and the Fear Driving the Greatest Scientific, Political, and Religious Debate of Our Time.* New York: Amacom, 2006.

Leo Furcht and William Hoffman, *The Stem Cell Debate: Beacons of Hope or Harbingers of Doom?* New York: Arcade, 2008.

Eve Herold, *Stem Cell Wars: Inside Stories from the Frontlines.* New York: Palgrave Macmillan, 2006.

Russell Korobkin, *Stem Cell Century: Law and Policy for a Breakthrough Technology.* New Haven, CT: Yale University Press, 2009.

Ed Regis, *What Is Life? Investigating the Nature of Life in the Age of Synthetic Biology.* New York: Oxford University Press USA, 2009.

Jennifer L. Skancke, ed., *Stem Cell Research: Opposing Viewpoints.* Farmington Hills, MI: Greenhaven, 2009.

Clive Niels Svendsen and Allison D. Ebert, eds., *Encyclopedia of Stem Cell Research.* Thousand Oaks, CA: Sage, 2008.

Lisa Yount, *Biotechnology and Genetic Engineering: Library in a Book.* New York: Facts On File, 2008.

Periodicals

Barbara Basler, "Brain Cancer: Could Adult Stem Cells Be the Cause—and the Cure?" *AARP Bulletin Today*, November 1, 2008.

Eric Cohen, "Celling Spin: The Reasonableness of the Bush Policy, and the Unreasonableness of Its Critics," *National Review*, May 3, 2006.

Bernadine Healy, "A Stem Cell Victory: Human Stem Cells Now Can Be Made from Adult Skin, Without Using Embryos or Eggs," *U.S. News & World Report*, January 2, 2008.

Michael J. Sandel, "Embryo Ethics," *Boston Globe*, April 8, 2007.

Steven Thomma, "Ending 'War on Science,' Obama Allows Federal Financing on Research on Embryonic Stem Cells," *Pittsburgh Post-Gazette*, March 10, 2009.

Internet Sources

CNN, "President George W. Bush's Address on Stem Cell Research," August 9, 2001. http://archives.cnn.com/2001/ALL POLITICS/08/09/bush.transcript.

Erica Lloyd, "Umbilical Cord Blood: The Future of Stem Cell Research?" *National Geographic*, April 6, 2006. http://news.national geographic.com/news/2006/04/0406_060406_cord_blood.html.

Nova, "ScienceNow," PBS. www.pbs.org/wgbh/nova/sciencenow/dispatches/050413.html.

Washington Post, "On Faith: The (Im)Morality of Stem Cell Research." http://newsweek.washingtonpost.com/onfaith/2009/03/embryonic_stem_cell_research/all.html.

The White House, "Removing Barriers to Responsible Scientific Research Involving Human Stem Cells," March 9, 2009. www.whitehouse.gov/the_press_office/Removing-Barriers-to-Responsible-Scientific-Research-Involving-Human-Stem-cells.

Web Sites

Stem Cells at the National Academies (http://dels.nas.edu/bls/stem cells). Maintained by the National Academies, the federal government's advisory agency on science, the Web site provides several reports, brochures, and booklets on stem cells, cloning, and genetic engineering that visitors can download.

Tell Me About Stem Cells (www.tellmeaboutstemcells.org). Written by professors at Harvard University Medical School and the Massachusetts Institute of Technology, this Web site includes some basic information about stem cells, walking readers through how stem cells form, how they change in the body, and which diseases they may be able to cure.

Source Notes

Introduction: Stem Cell Research: The Moral Debate

1. Quoted in *Anderson Cooper 360 Degrees*, "Interview with Michael J. Fox," CNN, November 5, 2006. http://transcripts.cnn.com.

2. Quoted in Standard News Wire, "Brownback Opposes Obama Stem Cell Policy," March 9, 2009. www.standardnewswire.com.

3. Quoted in Marie McCullough, "Scientists See Big Impact in Obama Move," *Philadelphia Inquirer*, March 10, 2009, p. A-1.

4. Quoted in *BusinessWeek*, "Michael J. Fox's Take on Stem Cells," May 24, 2004. www.businessweek.com.

Chapter One: What Are the Origins of the Stem Cell Controversy?

5. Quoted in Howard M. Lenhoff and Sylvia G. Lenhoff, *A History of Regeneration Research: Milestones in the Evolution of Science.* Cambridge, England: Cambridge University Press, 1991, p. 56.

6. Quoted in Lenhoff and Lenhoff, *A History of Regeneration Research*, p. 107.

7. Eve Herold, "Stem Cells and the Future of Medicine," *USA Today*, March 2003, p. 56.

8. Quoted in Kyla Dunn, "The Politics of Stem Cells," *Nova*, April 13, 2005. www.pbs.org.

9. Quoted in CNN, "President George W. Bush's Address on Stem Cell Research," August 9, 2001. http://archives.cnn.com.

10. Quoted in CBS News, "Arlen Specter's Stem Cell Battle," June 3, 2005. www.cbsnews.com.

11. Quoted in Associated Press, "Stem Cell Debate Moves to Senate," MSNBC, May 25, 2005. www.msnbc.msn.com.

12. Quoted in Nancy Gibbs, Alice Park, and Dan Cray, "Stem Cells: The Hope and the Hype," *Time*, August 7, 2006, p. 40.

13. Senator Robert Menendez, "Citing Painful Connection to Alzheimer's, Senator Urges Stem Cell Research," April 10, 2007. http://menendez.senate.gov.

14. Quoted in Harvard Stem Cell Institute, "CAMR Poll: Nearly Three-Quarters of Americans Support Embryonic Stem Cell Research," May 16, 2006. www.hsci.harvard.edu.

15. Quoted in Steven Thomma, "Ending 'War on Science,' Obama Allows Federal Financing on Research on Embryonic Stem Cells," *Pittsburgh Post-Gazette*, March 10, 2009, p. A-4.

Chapter Two: What Benefits Could Stem Cell Research Offer?

16. Quoted in *Stem Cell Week*, "Batten Disease: Historic Breakthrough in Fighting Childhood Batten Disease as China Stem Cells Give New Lease on Life to 6-Year-Old California Boy," February 11, 2008, p. 90.

17. Quoted in Peter Korn, "A Stem Cell First at OHSU," *Portland Tribune*, November 24, 2006. www.portlandtribune.com.

18. Peter Aldhous, "Miracle Postponed: In the Light of the Korean Scandal, Many Big Claims About Stem Cells Are Looking Decidedly Doubtful," *New Scientist*, March 11, 2006, p. 38.

19. Quoted in Paul Elias, Associated Press, "Child Who Received Stem Cells from Aborted Fetus on the Way Home," *Sign On San Diego*, December 12, 2006. www.signonsandiego.com.

20. Senator Barbara A. Mikulski, "Stem Cell Research Is About Saving Lives, Not Party Lines," April 11, 2007. http://mikulski.senate.gov.

21. Religious Action Center of Reform Judaism, "Stem Cell Research," July 26, 2005. http://rac.org.

22. Quoted in Roxanne Patel Shepelavy, "How Far Would You Go for a Cure?" MSNBC, March 9, 2008. www.msnbc.msn.com.

23. Quoted in Shepelavy, "How Far Would You Go for a Cure?"

24. Quoted in Nicki Lefever, "Saving Shawna: A Search for Hope," *York Daily Record*, August 25, 2008. http://ydr.inyork.com.

25. Quoted in CNN, "Scientists: Rats Partially Overcome Paralysis in Stem Cell Study," June 22, 2006. www.cnn.com.

26. Marcus Grompe, "Alternative Energy for Embryonic Stem Cell Research," *Nature Reports*, October 11, 2007. www.nature.com.

27. Judie Brown, "We Deserve Better than Embryonic Stem Cell Research Fraud," *Renew America*, January 10, 2007. www.renew america.us.

28. Quoted in Brandon Keim, "Stem Cell Tumor a Cautionary Reminder," *Wired*, February 18, 2009. http://blog.wired.com.

29. Quoted in Nikhili Swaminathan, "Body May Reject Transplanted Human Embryonic Stem Cells," *Scientific American*, August 19, 2008. www.sciam.com.

30. David A. Prentice, Family Research Council, testimony before the Mississippi Senate Public Health and Welfare Committee, February 22, 2006. www.stemcellresearch.org.

31. Robert Winston, "Should We Trust the Scientists?" Gresham College, June 20, 2005. www.gresham.ac.uk.

32. Elizabeth G. Phimister and Jeffrey M. Drazen, "Two Fillips for Human Embryonic Stem Cells," *New England Journal of Medicine*, March 25, 2004, p. 1,351.

33. Quoted in Choe Sang-Hun and Nicholas Wade, "Korean Cloning Scientist Quits over Report He Faked Research," *New York Times*, December 24, 2005, A-1.

34. Herold, "Stem Cells and the Future of Medicine," p. 58.

Chapter Three: Should Scientific Promise Outweigh Moral Concerns?

35. David P. Gushee, "The Stem-Cell Veto," Center for Bioethics and Human Dignity, July 20, 2006. www.cbhd.org.

36. Rosemary Radford Ruether, "'Consistent Life Ethic' Is Inconsistent," *National Catholic Reporter*, November 17, 2006, p. 13.

37. Quoted in Associated Press, "Obama Says He Was Too Flip on Abortion Issue," MSNBC, September 7, 2008. www.msnbc.msn.com.

38. Robert P. George, "A Distinct Human Organism," National Public Radio, November 22, 2005. www.npr.org.

39. David Holcberg and Alex Epstein, "The Anti-Life Opposition to Embryonic Stem Cell Research," *Northwest Arkansas Times*, May 31, 2005. www.nwanews.com.

40. Michael J. Sandel, "Embryo Ethics—the Moral Logic of Stem-Cell Research," *New England Journal of Medicine*, July 15, 2004, p. 208.

41. Michael J. Sandel, "Embryo Ethics," *Boston Globe*, April 8, 2007. www.boston.com.

42. Menendez, "Citing Painful Connection to Alzheimer's, Senator Urges Stem Cell Research."

43. Holcberg and Epstein, "The Anti-Life Opposition to Embryonic Stem Cell Research."

44. William J. Saunders, Testimony in Support of "Human Cloning Prohibition Act of 2006," Before the Health and Government Operations Committee of the Maryland House of Delegates, March 17, 2006. www.stemcellresearch.org.

45. Gushee, "The Stem-Cell Veto."

46. Brown, "We Deserve Better than Embryonic Stem Cell Research Fraud."

47. Quoted in W. Reed Moran, "Mary Tyler Moore Lobbies for Diabetes Research," *USA Today*, July 9, 2001. www.usatoday.com.

48. Saunders, Testimony in Support of "Human Cloning Prohibition Act of 2006."

49. Saunders, Testimony in Support of "Human Cloning Prohibition Act of 2006."

50. Alex Epstein, "The Religious Right's Culture of Living Death," *Capitalism*, April 29, 2007. www.capmag.com.

Chapter Four: Are There Effective Alternatives to Embryonic Stem Cell Research?

51. Quoted in CNN, "Adult Stem Cells or Embryonic? Scientists Differ," August 9, 2001. http://transcripts.cnn.com.

52. Wolfgang Lillge, "The Case for Adult Stem Cell Research," *21st Century*, Winter 2001–2002. www.21stcenturysciencetech.com.

53. Jean Peduzzi-Nelson, "Adult Stem Cells Are Behind Much of Stem Cell Success So Far," *Milwaukee Journal Sentinel*, September 3, 2006.

54. Quoted in CNN, "Adult Stem Cells or Embryonic? Scientists Differ."

55. Wesley J. Smith, "The Great Stem Cell Coverup," *Weekly Standard*, August 7, 2006. www.weeklystandard.com.

56. Quoted in University of Pittsburgh McGowan Institute for Regenerative Medicine, "Adult Stem Cell Injections in Heart Failure Patients Show Treatment's Benefit," news release, April 25, 2004. www.mirm.pitt.edu.

57. Quoted in Nikki Buskey, "Medicinal Miracle Saves Man's Heart," *Houma Today*, March 15, 2009. www.houmatoday.com.

58. Quoted in Buskey, "Medicinal Miracle Saves Man's Heart."

59. Quoted in Medical News Today, "Combination Adult Stem Cell Therapy Improves Severe Limb Ischemia," April 2, 2009. www.medicalnewstoday.com.

60. Quoted in *Innovation*, "Miracle Cell," April 13, 2004. www.pbs.org.

61. Quoted in *Innovation*, "Miracle Cell."

62. Quoted in CNN, "Adult Stem Cells or Embryonic? Scientists Differ."

63. Quoted in Barbara Basler, "Brain Cancer: Could Adult Stem Cells Be the Cause—and the Cure?" *AARP Bulletin Today*, November 1, 2008. http://bulletin.aarp.org.

64. Quoted in CNN, "Adult Stem Cells or Embryonic? Scientists Differ."

65. Bernadine Healy, "A Stem Cell Victory: Human Stem Cells Now Can Be Made from Adult Skin, Without Using Embryos or Eggs," *U.S. News & World Report*, January 2, 2008. http://health.usnews.com.

66. Thomas G. Bohlin, "Why Destroy Life? We Have Better Alternatives," *Washington Post*, March 10, 2009. http://newsweek.washingtonpost.com.

67. Quoted in *Nature*, "Stem Cells: A New Path to Pluripotency," February 14, 2008. www.nature.com.

68. Healy, "A Stem Cell Victory."

69. Healy, "A Stem Cell Victory."

Chapter Five: Should the Government Support Stem Cell Research?

70. Quoted in The White House, "President Discusses Embryo Adoption and Ethical Stem Cell Research," May 24, 2005. www.whitehouse.gov.

71. Quoted in Ceci Connolly, "Compromise Rules Issued on Embryonic Stem Cells," *Washington Post*, April 18, 2009. www.washingtonpost.com.

72. Quoted in Alice Park, "NIH Eases Restrictions on Stem Cells," *Time*, April 17, 2009. www.time.com.

73. Quoted in Connolly, "Compromise Rules Issued on Embryonic Stem Cells."

74. Quoted in Gardiner Harris, "Some Stem Cell Research Limits Lifted," *New York Times*, April 17, 2009. www.nytimes.com.

75. Eric Cohen, "Celling Spin: The Reasonableness of the Bush Policy, and the Unreasonableness of Its Critics," *National Review*, May 3, 2006. http://article.nationalreview.com.

76. Quoted in Steven Edwards, "Scrutinizing a Stem Cell Trial," *Wired*, March 29, 2006. www.wired.com.

77. Jennifer McCormick and Jason Owen-Smith, "An International Gap in Human ES Cell Research," *Nature Biotechnology*, April 2006, p. 392.

78. Mikulski, "Stem Cell Research Is About Saving Lives, Not Party Lines."

79. Mikulski, "Stem Cell Research Is About Saving Lives, Not Party Lines."

80. Quoted in Todd Finkelmeyer, "Controversial 'Stem Cell Tourism' Attracts Ailing Americans," *Madison (WI) Capital Times*, September 23, 2008. www.madison.com.

81. Quoted in Finkelmeyer, "Controversial 'Stem Cell Tourism' Attracts Ailing Americans."

82. Quoted in *Gulf Times*, "Stem Cell Transplant for Eye Repair Raises Concern," January 18, 2007. www.gulf-times.com.

83. Quoted in *Gulf Times*, "Stem Cell Transplant for Eye Repair Raises Concern."

84. Quoted in Lea Winerman, "States Move to Restrict Stem Cell Research After Obama Lifts Federal Restriction," Online News Hour, April 3, 2009. www.pbs.org.

Index

adult stem cell research, support for, 62–64
adult stem cells, 15
  advantages of, 55
  disadvantages of, 56, 62
  potential dangers of, 61–62
  sources of, 54, 59 (illustration)
  in treatment of heart disease, 58, 60, 65
  in treatment of HIV/AIDS, 57
Aldhous, Peter, 26
Alzheimer's disease, 38
Amerson, Amos, 79

Baetge, Ed, 68
Batten's disease, 24, 25, 38
Bavister, Barry, 16
blastocysts, 9, 12–13
  ethical debate over destruction of, 39–45
Blau, Helen, 53–54, 62
Bohlin, Thomas G., 64
bone marrow transplants, first, 15
Brown, Judie, 33, 48
Brownback, Sam, 8
Bush, George H.W., 18
Bush, George W., 20, 23, 40, 42, 66–67

cancer, risk of treating, with adult stem cells, 62
Cathcart, Aaron, 58, 60
cells, somatic vs. germ, 12
Charo, R. Alta, 69
Clinton, Bill, 18, 19
cloning. *See* reproductive cloning; therapeutic cloning
Coalition for the Advancement of Medical research, 23
Cohen, Eric, 70
Corzine, Jon, 73

Daley, George, 64
Darwin, Charles, 47
Dell'Arriga, Blake, 24–25, 26, 28
Department of Health and Human Services, U.S. (HHS), 18
diabetes, 38
  stem cells as potential cure for, 30
Dickey, Jay, 18, 19
Dickey-Wicker Amendment (1995), 19
DNA, 35, 62, 63
  scientists' ability to alter, 38
Dolly (cloned sheep), 52
Dominguez, Laura, 61
Drazen, Jeffrey M., 34

Edwards, Robert, 15–16
embryonic stem cell research
  complexity of, 33–34
  cost of, 66
  effects of economic downturn on, 73
  federal funding of, 9–10
    ban on, 17–18, 20
    NIH issues guidelines for, 67–69
    public support for, 69–70
    role of Congress in, 79
  obstacles created by federal ban on funding of, 19
  opposition to, 8
  risk of U.S. falling behind in, 72–74
  state policies on, 78 (map)
  states funding, 77
  support for, 9, 65
embryonic stem cells
  pluripotent nature of, 27–28
  as treatment of heart disease, 65
Epstein, Alex, 43–44, 46, 51
Ethics & Public Policy Center, 47
eugenics, 47

Food and Drug Administration, U.S. (FDA), first stem cell test approved by, 68
Fox, Michael J., 6–7, 10
Furlanetto, Richard, 49

Galton, Francis, 47
George, Robert P., 42–43
Geron Corporation, 68, 71
Grompe, Marcus, 33
Grumet, Martin, 73
Gushee, David P., 39, 48

Häcker, Valentin, 13
Healy, Bernadine, 63, 64–65
heart disease
    adult stem cells in treatment of, 58, 60, 65
    embryonic stem cells as treatment of, 65
Herold, Eve, 17, 37
HIV/AIDS, adult stem cells in treatment of, 57
Holcberg, David, 43–44, 46
Human Fetal Tissue Transplantation Research Panel, 18
Hutter, Gero, 57
Hwang Woo Suk, 36–37
hydra, 11

in vitro fertilization, 15–16, 42
in vitro fertilization clinics
    number of children born from embryos stored in, 52
    number of embryos destroyed annually, 23
    number of frozen blastocysts stored at, 16
    as source for embryonic stem cells, 9, 10

Jaeger, Jeremy, 24–25
Kim, Je Eun, 37
John Paul II (pope), 52
Johnson, Douglas, 70
Jülich Research Center, 79

Kerr, Douglas, 32

Kilgore, Ricci, 29–31
Kington, Raynard, 69

Lasala, Gabriel, 60
Lillge, Wolfgang, 55
Lima, Carlos, 60–61
liver, artificial, growth from stem cells, 27
lower limb ischemia, treatment with adult stem cells, 60–61

McCain, John, 22
McCormick, Jennifer, 72
McCulloch, Earnest A., 15
Melton, Douglas, 21
Menendez, Robert, 21, 45
Mikulski, Barbara A., 28, 73–74
miscarriage, 44
Moore, Mary Tyler, 30
Moreno, Jonathan, 19
Morgan, Thomas Hunt, 13–15

National Institutes of Health (NIH), 18, 56
    issues guidelines on for federally funded stem cell research, 67–69
Nature Biotechnology (journal), 72, 79
Nuremberg Code, 47–48

Obama, Barack, 9, 14, 40, 67
    on scientific research and politics, 22
Okarma, Tom, 71
O'Malley, Martin, 73
organ transplantation, 38
organogenesis, 27, 28
Owen-Smith, Jason, 72

Parkinson's disease (PD), 6, 50
    percent affected under 40 years of age, 10
Patel, Amit, 58
Peduzzi-Nelson, Jean, 55
Phimister, Elizabeth G., 34
Prentice, David A., 34, 63

Quiñones-Hinojosa, Alfredo, 62

Rader, William, 29
Reagan, Nancy, 23
Reagan, Ronald, 23
Reeve, Christopher, 14
Religious Action Center of Reform
    Judaism, 28
reproductive cloning, 8, 49
    animals born from, 52
research. *See* adult stem cell research;
    embryonic stem cell research
Reynolds, Mike, 77
Roe v. Wade (1973), 18
Rosen, Christine, 47
Ruether, Rosemary Radford, 39

Sandel, Michael J., 44–45
Saunders, William J., 47, 49, 51
Science (journal), 23
Shalala, Donna, 18
Sinden, John, 73
Smith, Wesley J., 56–57
snowflake children, 42
Solomon, Susan L., 69
somatic cell nuclear transfer (SCNT).
    See therapeutic cloning
Specter, Arlen, 20
Steiner, Robert, 26
stem cell lines
    creation of, 16–17
    number approved for federal
        funding, 21
    number potentially created from
        frozen embryos, 38
    pre-2001, problems with, 71
stem cell niches, 54
stem cell therapy
    Americans traveling abroad to
        receive, 28–32
        lifting federal ban on funding
            may reverse, 74–77
    diseases potentially treated by, 17
    potential of, may take years to
        realize, 77–79
stem cells
    creation of, 25 (illustration)

See also adult stem cells; embryonic
    stem cells
Sullivan, Louis, 18
surveys
    on federally funded stem cell
        research, 69–70
    on importance of curing human
        disease vs. protecting life of
        embryo, 46
    of infertile couples on willingness to
        donate excess embryos, 23
    on promise of embryonic vs. adult
        stem cell research, 65
    on stem cell research and religion,
        40
    on stem cell research involving
        destruction of embryo, 44
    on use of human cloning to develop
        cures for disease, 52
    on use of human embryos in
        research, 10, 21, 23

Tabar, Viviane, 50
therapeutic cloning (somatic cell
    nuclear transfer), 34–36
    guidelines would ensure responsible
        use of, 51
    opposition to, 48–50
    scandal in South Korea over,
        36–37
Till, James E., 15
Time (magazine), 21
Tipton, Sean, 21–22, 25
Trembley, Abraham, 11–12

umbilical cord blood, 54–55
United States, risks falling behind
    other nations in stem cell research,
    72–74, 79

Weil, Shawna, 31
Wicker, Roger, 19
Winston, Robert, 34
Wu, Joseph, 34

25.95   4/14/10